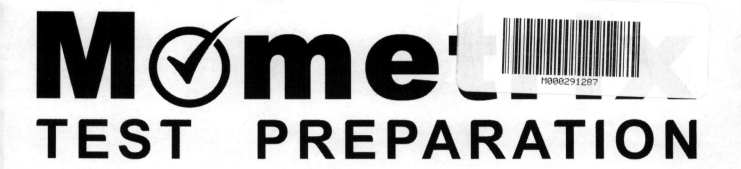

TEST PREPARATION

CMC
Exam Secrets
Study Guide

DEAR FUTURE EXAM SUCCESS STORY

First of all, **THANK YOU** for purchasing Mometrix study materials!

Second, congratulations! You are one of the few determined test-takers who are committed to doing whatever it takes to excel on your exam. **You have come to the right place.** We developed these study materials with one goal in mind: to deliver you the information you need in a format that's concise and easy to use.

In addition to optimizing your guide for the content of the test, we've outlined our recommended steps for breaking down the preparation process into small, attainable goals so you can make sure you stay on track.

We've also analyzed the entire test-taking process, identifying the most common pitfalls and showing how you can overcome them and be ready for any curveball the test throws you.

Standardized testing is one of the biggest obstacles on your road to success, which only increases the importance of doing well in the high-pressure, high-stakes environment of test day. Your results on this test could have a significant impact on your future, and this guide provides the information and practical advice to help you achieve your full potential on test day.

Your success is our success

We would love to hear from you! If you would like to share the story of your exam success or if you have any questions or comments in regard to our products, please contact us at **800-673-8175** or **support@mometrix.com**.

Thanks again for your business and we wish you continued success!

Sincerely,
The Mometrix Test Preparation Team

Need more help? Check out our flashcards at:
http://mometrixflashcards.com/CMC

TABLE OF CONTENTS

Introduction

Thank you for purchasing this resource! You have made the choice to prepare yourself for a test that could have a huge impact on your future, and this guide is designed to help you be fully ready for test day. Obviously, it's important to have a solid understanding of the test material, but you also need to be prepared for the unique environment and stressors of the test, so that you can perform to the best of your abilities.

For this purpose, the first section that appears in this guide is the **Secret Keys**. We've devoted countless hours to meticulously researching what works and what doesn't, and we've boiled down our findings to the five most impactful steps you can take to improve your performance on the test. We start at the beginning with study planning and move through the preparation process, all the way to the testing strategies that will help you get the most out of what you know when you're finally sitting in front of the test.

We recommend that you start preparing for your test as far in advance as possible. However, if you've bought this guide as a last-minute study resource and only have a few days before your test, we recommend that you skip over the first two Secret Keys since they address a long-term study plan.

If you struggle with **test anxiety**, we strongly encourage you to check out our recommendations for how you can overcome it. Test anxiety is a formidable foe, but it can be beaten, and we want to make sure you have the tools you need to defeat it.

Secret Key #1 – Plan Big, Study Small

There's a lot riding on your performance. If you want to ace this test, you're going to need to keep your skills sharp and the material fresh in your mind. You need a plan that lets you review everything you need to know while still fitting in your schedule. We'll break this strategy down into three categories.

Information Organization

Start with the information you already have: the official test outline. From this, you can make a complete list of all the concepts you need to cover before the test. Organize these concepts into groups that can be studied together, and create a list of any related vocabulary you need to learn so you can brush up on any difficult terms. You'll want to keep this vocabulary list handy once you actually start studying since you may need to add to it along the way.

Time Management

Once you have your set of study concepts, decide how to spread them out over the time you have left before the test. Break your study plan into small, clear goals so you have a manageable task for each day and know exactly what you're doing. Then just focus on one small step at a time. When you manage your time this way, you don't need to spend hours at a time studying. Studying a small block of content for a short period each day helps you retain information better and avoid stressing over how much you have left to do. You can relax knowing that you have a plan to cover everything in time. In order for this strategy to be effective though, you have to start studying early and stick to your schedule. Avoid the exhaustion and futility that comes from last-minute cramming!

Study Environment

The environment you study in has a big impact on your learning. Studying in a coffee shop, while probably more enjoyable, is not likely to be as fruitful as studying in a quiet room. It's important to keep distractions to a minimum. You're only planning to study for a short block of time, so make the most of it. Don't pause to check your phone or get up to find a snack. It's also important to **avoid multitasking**. Research has consistently shown that multitasking will make your studying dramatically less effective. Your study area should also be comfortable and well-lit so you don't have the distraction of straining your eyes or sitting on an uncomfortable chair.

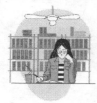 The time of day you study is also important. You want to be rested and alert. Don't wait until just before bedtime. Study when you'll be most likely to comprehend and remember. Even better, if you know what time of day your test will be, set that time aside for study. That way your brain will be used to working on that subject at that specific time and you'll have a better chance of recalling information.

Finally, it can be helpful to team up with others who are studying for the same test. Your actual studying should be done in as isolated an environment as possible, but the work of organizing the information and setting up the study plan can be divided up. In between study sessions, you can discuss with your teammates the concepts that you're all studying and quiz each other on the details. Just be sure that your teammates are as serious about the test as you are. If you find that your study time is being replaced with social time, you might need to find a new team.

Secret Key #2 – Make Your Studying Count

You're devoting a lot of time and effort to preparing for this test, so you want to be absolutely certain it will pay off. This means doing more than just reading the content and hoping you can remember it on test day. It's important to make every minute of study count. There are two main areas you can focus on to make your studying count.

Retention

It doesn't matter how much time you study if you can't remember the material. You need to make sure you are retaining the concepts. To check your retention of the information you're learning, try recalling it at later times with minimal prompting. Try carrying around flashcards and glance at one or two from time to time or ask a friend who's also studying for the test to quiz you.

To enhance your retention, look for ways to put the information into practice so that you can apply it rather than simply recalling it. If you're using the information in practical ways, it will be much easier to remember. Similarly, it helps to solidify a concept in your mind if you're not only reading it to yourself but also explaining it to someone else. Ask a friend to let you teach them about a concept you're a little shaky on (or speak aloud to an imaginary audience if necessary). As you try to summarize, define, give examples, and answer your friend's questions, you'll understand the concepts better and they will stay with you longer. Finally, step back for a big picture view and ask yourself how each piece of information fits with the whole subject. When you link the different concepts together and see them working together as a whole, it's easier to remember the individual components.

Finally, practice showing your work on any multi-step problems, even if you're just studying. Writing out each step you take to solve a problem will help solidify the process in your mind, and you'll be more likely to remember it during the test.

Modality

Modality simply refers to the means or method by which you study. Choosing a study modality that fits your own individual learning style is crucial. No two people learn best in exactly the same way, so it's important to know your strengths and use them to your advantage.

For example, if you learn best by visualization, focus on visualizing a concept in your mind and draw an image or a diagram. Try color-coding your notes, illustrating them, or creating symbols that will trigger your mind to recall a learned concept. If you learn best by hearing or discussing information, find a study partner who learns the same way or read aloud to yourself. Think about how to put the information in your own words. Imagine that you are giving a lecture on the topic and record yourself so you can listen to it later.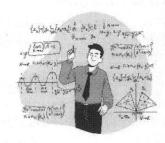

For any learning style, flashcards can be helpful. Organize the information so you can take advantage of spare moments to review. Underline key words or phrases. Use different colors for different categories. Mnemonic devices (such as creating a short list in which every item starts with the same letter) can also help with retention. Find what works best for you and use it to store the information in your mind most effectively and easily.

3

Secret Key #3 – Practice the Right Way

Your success on test day depends not only on how many hours you put into preparing, but also on whether you prepared the right way. It's good to check along the way to see if your studying is paying off. One of the most effective ways to do this is by taking practice tests to evaluate your progress. Practice tests are useful because they show exactly where you need to improve. Every time you take a practice test, pay special attention to these three groups of questions:

- The questions you got wrong
- The questions you had to guess on, even if you guessed right
- The questions you found difficult or slow to work through

This will show you exactly what your weak areas are, and where you need to devote more study time. Ask yourself why each of these questions gave you trouble. Was it because you didn't understand the material? Was it because you didn't remember the vocabulary? Do you need more repetitions on this type of question to build speed and confidence? Dig into those questions and figure out how you can strengthen your weak areas as you go back to review the material.

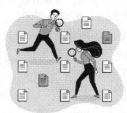 Additionally, many practice tests have a section explaining the answer choices. It can be tempting to read the explanation and think that you now have a good understanding of the concept. However, an explanation likely only covers part of the question's broader context. Even if the explanation makes perfect sense, **go back and investigate** every concept related to the question until you're positive you have a thorough understanding.

As you go along, keep in mind that the practice test is just that: practice. Memorizing these questions and answers will not be very helpful on the actual test because it is unlikely to have any of the same exact questions. If you only know the right answers to the sample questions, you won't be prepared for the real thing. **Study the concepts** until you understand them fully, and then you'll be able to answer any question that shows up on the test.

It's important to wait on the practice tests until you're ready. If you take a test on your first day of study, you may be overwhelmed by the amount of material covered and how much you need to learn. Work up to it gradually.

On test day, you'll need to be prepared for answering questions, managing your time, and using the test-taking strategies you've learned. It's a lot to balance, like a mental marathon that will have a big impact on your future. Like training for a marathon, you'll need to start slowly and work your way up. When test day arrives, you'll be ready.

Start with the strategies you've read in the first two Secret Keys—plan your course and study in the way that works best for you. If you have time, consider using multiple study resources to get different approaches to the same concepts. It can be helpful to see difficult concepts from more than one angle. Then find a good source for practice tests. Many times, the test website will suggest potential study resources or provide sample tests.

Practice Test Strategy

If you're able to find at least three practice tests, we recommend this strategy:

UNTIMED AND OPEN-BOOK PRACTICE

Take the first test with no time constraints and with your notes and study guide handy. Take your time and focus on applying the strategies you've learned.

TIMED AND OPEN-BOOK PRACTICE

Take the second practice test open-book as well, but set a timer and practice pacing yourself to finish in time.

TIMED AND CLOSED-BOOK PRACTICE

Take any other practice tests as if it were test day. Set a timer and put away your study materials. Sit at a table or desk in a quiet room, imagine yourself at the testing center, and answer questions as quickly and accurately as possible.

Keep repeating timed and closed-book tests on a regular basis until you run out of practice tests or it's time for the actual test. Your mind will be ready for the schedule and stress of test day, and you'll be able to focus on recalling the material you've learned.

Secret Key #4 – Pace Yourself

Once you're fully prepared for the material on the test, your biggest challenge on test day will be managing your time. Just knowing that the clock is ticking can make you panic even if you have plenty of time left. Work on pacing yourself so you can build confidence against the time constraints of the exam. Pacing is a difficult skill to master, especially in a high-pressure environment, so **practice is vital**.

Set time expectations for your pace based on how much time is available. For example, if a section has 60 questions and the time limit is 30 minutes, you know you have to average 30 seconds or less per question in order to answer them all. Although 30 seconds is the hard limit, set 25 seconds per question as your goal, so you reserve extra time to spend on harder questions. When you budget extra time for the harder questions, you no longer have any reason to stress when those questions take longer to answer.

Don't let this time expectation distract you from working through the test at a calm, steady pace, but keep it in mind so you don't spend too much time on any one question. Recognize that taking extra time on one question you don't understand may keep you from answering two that you do understand later in the test. If your time limit for a question is up and you're still not sure of the answer, mark it and move on, and come back to it later if the time and the test format allow. If the testing format doesn't allow you to return to earlier questions, just make an educated guess; then put it out of your mind and move on.

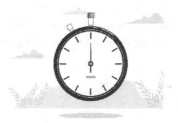

On the easier questions, be careful not to rush. It may seem wise to hurry through them so you have more time for the challenging ones, but it's not worth missing one if you know the concept and just didn't take the time to read the question fully. Work efficiently but make sure you understand the question and have looked at all of the answer choices, since more than one may seem right at first.

Even if you're paying attention to the time, you may find yourself a little behind at some point. You should speed up to get back on track, but do so wisely. Don't panic; just take a few seconds less on each question until you're caught up. Don't guess without thinking, but do look through the answer choices and eliminate any you know are wrong. If you can get down to two choices, it is often worthwhile to guess from those. Once you've chosen an answer, move on and don't dwell on any that you skipped or had to hurry through. If a question was taking too long, chances are it was one of the harder ones, so you weren't as likely to get it right anyway.

On the other hand, if you find yourself getting ahead of schedule, it may be beneficial to slow down a little. The more quickly you work, the more likely you are to make a careless mistake that will affect your score. You've budgeted time for each question, so don't be afraid to spend that time. Practice an efficient but careful pace to get the most out of the time you have.

6

Secret Key #5 – Have a Plan for Guessing

When you're taking the test, you may find yourself stuck on a question. Some of the answer choices seem better than others, but you don't see the one answer choice that is obviously correct. What do you do?

The scenario described above is very common, yet most test takers have not effectively prepared for it. Developing and practicing a plan for guessing may be one of the single most effective uses of your time as you get ready for the exam.

In developing your plan for guessing, there are three questions to address:

- When should you start the guessing process?
- How should you narrow down the choices?
- Which answer should you choose?

When to Start the Guessing Process

Unless your plan for guessing is to select C every time (which, despite its merits, is not what we recommend), you need to leave yourself enough time to apply your answer elimination strategies. Since you have a limited amount of time for each question, that means that if you're going to give yourself the best shot at guessing correctly, you have to decide quickly whether or not you will guess.

Of course, the best-case scenario is that you don't have to guess at all, so first, see if you can answer the question based on your knowledge of the subject and basic reasoning skills. Focus on the key words in the question and try to jog your memory of related topics. Give yourself a chance to bring the knowledge to mind, but once you realize that you don't have (or you can't access) the knowledge you need to answer the question, it's time to start the guessing process.

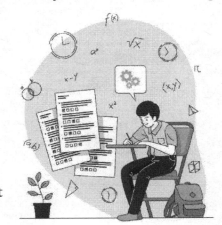

It's almost always better to start the guessing process too early than too late. It only takes a few seconds to remember something and answer the question from knowledge. Carefully eliminating wrong answer choices takes longer. Plus, going through the process of eliminating answer choices can actually help jog your memory.

Summary: Start the guessing process as soon as you decide that you can't answer the question based on your knowledge.

7

How to Narrow Down the Choices

The next chapter in this book (**Test-Taking Strategies**) includes a wide range of strategies for how to approach questions and how to look for answer choices to eliminate. You will definitely want to read those carefully, practice them, and figure out which ones work best for you. Here though, we're going to address a mindset rather than a particular strategy.

Your odds of guessing an answer correctly depend on how many options you are choosing from.

Number of options left	5	4	3	2	1
Odds of guessing correctly	20%	25%	33%	50%	100%

You can see from this chart just how valuable it is to be able to eliminate incorrect answers and make an educated guess, but there are two things that many test takers do that cause them to miss out on the benefits of guessing:

- Accidentally eliminating the correct answer
- Selecting an answer based on an impression

We'll look at the first one here, and the second one in the next section.

To avoid accidentally eliminating the correct answer, we recommend a thought exercise called **the $5 challenge**. In this challenge, you only eliminate an answer choice from contention if you are willing to bet $5 on it being wrong. Why $5? Five dollars is a small but not insignificant amount of money. It's an amount you could afford to lose but wouldn't want to throw away. And while losing

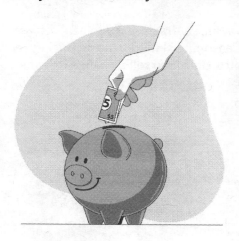

$5 once might not hurt too much, doing it twenty times will set you back $100. In the same way, each small decision you make—eliminating a choice here, guessing on a question there—won't by itself impact your score very much, but when you put them all together, they can make a big difference. By holding each answer choice elimination decision to a higher standard, you can reduce the risk of accidentally eliminating the correct answer.

The $5 challenge can also be applied in a positive sense: If you are willing to bet $5 that an answer choice *is* correct, go ahead and mark it as correct.

Summary: Only eliminate an answer choice if you are willing to bet $5 that it is wrong.

8

Which Answer to Choose

You're taking the test. You've run into a hard question and decided you'll have to guess. You've eliminated all the answer choices you're willing to bet $5 on. Now you have to pick an answer. Why do we even need to talk about this? Why can't you just pick whichever one you feel like when the time comes?

The answer to these questions is that if you don't come into the test with a plan, you'll rely on your impression to select an answer choice, and if you do that, you risk falling into a trap. The test writers know that everyone who takes their test will be guessing on some of the questions, so they intentionally write wrong answer choices to seem plausible. You still have to pick an answer though, and if the wrong answer choices are designed to look right, how can you ever be sure that you're not falling for their trap? The best solution we've found to this dilemma is to take the decision out of your hands entirely. Here is the process we recommend:

Once you've eliminated any choices that you are confident (willing to bet $5) are wrong, select the first remaining choice as your answer.

Whether you choose to select the first remaining choice, the second, or the last, the important thing is that you use some preselected standard. Using this approach guarantees that you will not be enticed into selecting an answer choice that looks right, because you are not basing your decision on how the answer choices look.

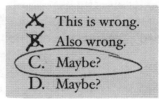

This is not meant to make you question your knowledge. Instead, it is to help you recognize the difference between your knowledge and your impressions. There's a huge difference between thinking an answer is right because of what you know, and thinking an answer is right because it looks or sounds like it should be right.

Summary: To ensure that your selection is appropriately random, make a predetermined selection from among all answer choices you have not eliminated.

Test-Taking Strategies

This section contains a list of test-taking strategies that you may find helpful as you work through the test. By taking what you know and applying logical thought, you can maximize your chances of answering any question correctly!

It is very important to realize that every question is different and every person is different: no single strategy will work on every question, and no single strategy will work for every person. That's why we've included all of them here, so you can try them out and determine which ones work best for different types of questions and which ones work best for you.

Question Strategies

⊘ READ CAREFULLY

Read the question and the answer choices carefully. Don't miss the question because you misread the terms. You have plenty of time to read each question thoroughly and make sure you understand what is being asked. Yet a happy medium must be attained, so don't waste too much time. You must read carefully and efficiently.

⊘ CONTEXTUAL CLUES

Look for contextual clues. If the question includes a word you are not familiar with, look at the immediate context for some indication of what the word might mean. Contextual clues can often give you all the information you need to decipher the meaning of an unfamiliar word. Even if you can't determine the meaning, you may be able to narrow down the possibilities enough to make a solid guess at the answer to the question.

⊘ PREFIXES

If you're having trouble with a word in the question or answer choices, try dissecting it. Take advantage of every clue that the word might include. Prefixes and suffixes can be a huge help. Usually, they allow you to determine a basic meaning. *Pre-* means before, *post-* means after, *pro-* is positive, *de-* is negative. From prefixes and suffixes, you can get an idea of the general meaning of the word and try to put it into context.

⊘ HEDGE WORDS

Watch out for critical hedge words, such as *likely, may, can, sometimes, often, almost, mostly, usually, generally, rarely,* and *sometimes.* Question writers insert these hedge phrases to cover every possibility. Often an answer choice will be wrong simply because it leaves no room for exception. Be on guard for answer choices that have definitive words such as *exactly* and *always.*

⊘ SWITCHBACK WORDS

Stay alert for *switchbacks.* These are the words and phrases frequently used to alert you to shifts in thought. The most common switchback words are *but, although,* and *however.* Others include *nevertheless, on the other hand, even though, while, in spite of, despite,* and *regardless of.* Switchback words are important to catch because they can change the direction of the question or an answer choice.

10

⏱ FACE VALUE

When in doubt, use common sense. Accept the situation in the problem at face value. Don't read too much into it. These problems will not require you to make wild assumptions. If you have to go beyond creativity and warp time or space in order to have an answer choice fit the question, then you should move on and consider the other answer choices. These are normal problems rooted in reality. The applicable relationship or explanation may not be readily apparent, but it is there for you to figure out. Use your common sense to interpret anything that isn't clear.

Answer Choice Strategies

⏱ ANSWER SELECTION

The most thorough way to pick an answer choice is to identify and eliminate wrong answers until only one is left, then confirm it is the correct answer. Sometimes an answer choice may immediately seem right, but be careful. The test writers will usually put more than one reasonable answer choice on each question, so take a second to read all of them and make sure that the other choices are not equally obvious. As long as you have time left, it is better to read every answer choice than to pick the first one that looks right without checking the others.

⏱ ANSWER CHOICE FAMILIES

An answer choice family consists of two (in rare cases, three) answer choices that are very similar in construction and cannot all be true at the same time. If you see two answer choices that are direct opposites or parallels, one of them is usually the correct answer. For instance, if one answer choice says that quantity x increases and another either says that quantity x decreases (opposite) or says that quantity y increases (parallel), then those answer choices would fall into the same family. An answer choice that doesn't match the construction of the answer choice family is more likely to be incorrect. Most questions will not have answer choice families, but when they do appear, you should be prepared to recognize them.

⏱ ELIMINATE ANSWERS

Eliminate answer choices as soon as you realize they are wrong, but make sure you consider all possibilities. If you are eliminating answer choices and realize that the last one you are left with is also wrong, don't panic. Start over and consider each choice again. There may be something you missed the first time that you will realize on the second pass.

⏱ AVOID FACT TRAPS

Don't be distracted by an answer choice that is factually true but doesn't answer the question. You are looking for the choice that answers the question. Stay focused on what the question is asking for so you don't accidentally pick an answer that is true but incorrect. Always go back to the question and make sure the answer choice you've selected actually answers the question and is not merely a true statement.

⏱ EXTREME STATEMENTS

In general, you should avoid answers that put forth extreme actions as standard practice or proclaim controversial ideas as established fact. An answer choice that states the "process should be used in certain situations, if..." is much more likely to be correct than one that states the "process should be discontinued completely." The first is a calm rational statement and doesn't even make a definitive, uncompromising stance, using a hedge word *if* to provide wiggle room, whereas the second choice is far more extreme.

☑ Benchmark

As you read through the answer choices and you come across one that seems to answer the question well, mentally select that answer choice. This is not your final answer, but it's the one that will help you evaluate the other answer choices. The one that you selected is your benchmark or standard for judging each of the other answer choices. Every other answer choice must be compared to your benchmark. That choice is correct until proven otherwise by another answer choice beating it. If you find a better answer, then that one becomes your new benchmark. Once you've decided that no other choice answers the question as well as your benchmark, you have your final answer.

☑ Predict the Answer

Before you even start looking at the answer choices, it is often best to try to predict the answer. When you come up with the answer on your own, it is easier to avoid distractions and traps because you will know exactly what to look for. The right answer choice is unlikely to be word-for-word what you came up with, but it should be a close match. Even if you are confident that you have the right answer, you should still take the time to read each option before moving on.

General Strategies

☑ Tough Questions

If you are stumped on a problem or it appears too hard or too difficult, don't waste time. Move on! Remember though, if you can quickly check for obviously incorrect answer choices, your chances of guessing correctly are greatly improved. Before you completely give up, at least try to knock out a couple of possible answers. Eliminate what you can and then guess at the remaining answer choices before moving on.

☑ Check Your Work

Since you will probably not know every term listed and the answer to every question, it is important that you get credit for the ones that you do know. Don't miss any questions through careless mistakes. If at all possible, try to take a second to look back over your answer selection and make sure you've selected the correct answer choice and haven't made a costly careless mistake (such as marking an answer choice that you didn't mean to mark). This quick double check should more than pay for itself in caught mistakes for the time it costs.

☑ Pace Yourself

It's easy to be overwhelmed when you're looking at a page full of questions; your mind is confused and full of random thoughts, and the clock is ticking down faster than you would like. Calm down and maintain the pace that you have set for yourself. Especially as you get down to the last few minutes of the test, don't let the small numbers on the clock make you panic. As long as you are on track by monitoring your pace, you are guaranteed to have time for each question.

☑ Don't Rush

It is very easy to make errors when you are in a hurry. Maintaining a fast pace in answering questions is pointless if it makes you miss questions that you would have gotten right otherwise. Test writers like to include distracting information and wrong answers that seem right. Taking a little extra time to avoid careless mistakes can make all the difference in your test score. Find a pace that allows you to be confident in the answers that you select.

12

⊘ KEEP MOVING

Panicking will not help you pass the test, so do your best to stay calm and keep moving. Taking deep breaths and going through the answer elimination steps you practiced can help to break through a stress barrier and keep your pace.

Final Notes

The combination of a solid foundation of content knowledge and the confidence that comes from practicing your plan for applying that knowledge is the key to maximizing your performance on test day. As your foundation of content knowledge is built up and strengthened, you'll find that the strategies included in this chapter become more and more effective in helping you quickly sift through the distractions and traps of the test to isolate the correct answer.

Now that you're preparing to move forward into the test content chapters of this book, be sure to keep your goal in mind. As you read, think about how you will be able to apply this information on the test. If you've already seen sample questions for the test and you have an idea of the question format and style, try to come up with questions of your own that you can answer based on what you're reading. This will give you valuable practice applying your knowledge in the same ways you can expect to on test day.

Good luck and good studying!

14

Cardiovascular Patient Care

Acute Coronary Syndrome

PATHOPHYSIOLOGY OF ACUTE CORONARY SYNDROME

Acute coronary syndrome (ACS) is an umbrella term used to cover any group of clinical symptoms resulting from acute myocardial ischemia. It often begins with the rupture of atherosclerotic plaque, creating an injured area on the endothelium. This results in platelet activation of the coagulation cascade and the formation of a thrombus over the injured area. The thrombus restricts blood flow to the cardiac muscle. Without the constant flow of oxygen-rich blood to the cardiac muscle, ischemia occurs. Cell injury and death secondary to cardiac ischemia cause the chest pain that is considered the most common symptom of ACS.

ACS is divided into three categories: unstable angina (USA), Non ST segment elevation MI (NSTEMI), and ST segment elevation MI (STEMI). Diagnosis of one of these categories is dependent upon the degree of cardiac muscle damage, the amount of time in which the coronary artery has been occluded, and the degree of occlusion.

UNSTABLE ANGINA, NON ST ELEVATION MI, AND ST ELEVATION MI

In the case of unstable angina (USA), there is no rise in cardiac biomarkers. If there is a decrease in left ventricular function secondary to cardiac ischemia, it returns to normal after the ischemia has resolved.

In cases of Non ST elevation MI there is no evidence of ST elevation. Cardiac biomarker levels will rise as a result of cardiac tissue injury, but the levels will not be high enough to render a positive test result. There may be some left ventricular dysfunction after a NSTEMI is corrected.

In a ST elevation MI, an ECG will show ST elevation. These elevations will be present in different leads depending upon where the injury is located. Further, depending on the severity of cardiac tissue damage, a Q wave may be present. CK-MB and troponin biomarkers are positive and there is a high risk for left ventricular dysfunction.

ACUTE CORONARY SYNDROME
RISK FACTORS

The primary risk factor for ACS is coronary artery disease, with the presence of atherosclerotic plaque on the walls of the arteries. CAD is present in all people, but the degree of plaque buildup is dependent on a number of risk factors. Some of these risk factors are manageable, and some are not.

Uncontrollable risk factors include age, gender and family history. A person's risk for CAD goes up if they are greater than 55 years old, and if they are male.

The controllable risk factors include smoking, obesity, hypercholesterolemia, hypertension, alcohol consumption, and a sedentary lifestyle. If a patient has been diagnosed with diabetes mellitus, their risk is higher if their blood sugar is uncontrolled.

Because of the myriad risk factors that affect the severity of CAD, it is important to obtain a complete medical history from the patient.

15

SIGNS AND SYMPTOMS

The most common symptom for acute coronary syndrome (ACS) is midsternal chest pain or pressure, which may radiate to the jaw or down the left arm. The patient may also present with nausea, vomiting, diaphoresis, shortness of breath, and a vague feeling of doom.

However, these symptoms are not universal. Some patients, particularly women and those with a prior history of diabetes may experience atypical symptoms such as localized pain in the neck, jaw, back or arms. They may complain of severe indigestion, sudden exhaustion or palpitations. Because the signs of ACS can be vague, it is important to acquire a complete medical history and perform a thorough assessment on all patients who display such symptoms.

ISCHEMIA, INJURY, INFARCTION, AND ECG CHANGES INVOLVED

Myocardial ischemia is the temporary slowing of blood flow to the myocardial tissue. Because the cardiac tissue is still getting some oxygenated blood, cellular death has not yet occurred. Myocardial ischemia is characterized by T-wave inversion on an ECG. Ischemic cells are still viable, and will return to a normal functioning when adequate blood flow is restored.

Injury occurs when there is prolonged interruption in the blood flow to the myocardial tissue. An elevated ST segment on an ECG characterizes cell injury.

Myocardial infarction occurs when there is no blood flow to an area of heart tissue. The cells involved in an infarction die and eventually necrose. They will be replaced by scar tissue after healing has occurred. Infarction is characterized by a Q wave duration of 0.04 seconds or longer. The Q wave will also be approximately one-fourth to one-third the height of the R wave.

ECG CHANGES PRESENT WHEN THE LATERAL, POSTERIOR, AND RIGHT VENTRICULAR WALLS ARE INVOLVED IN AN INFARCTION

When there are lead changes in I and aVL, it indicates a possible occlusion in the circumflex artery or a branch from the left anterior descending artery. Reciprocal changes may be seen in leads V_1 and V_3.

When the posterior wall is affected, ECG changes will be seen in leads V_1 and V_2, with reciprocal changes seen in leads V_1, V_2, V_3, and V_4. In leads V_1 and V_2, the R wave will be greater than the S wave. This indicates a possible occlusion in the right coronary artery or circumflex artery.

When there are lead changes in V_4, V_5, and V_6, it indicates involvement of the right ventricular wall. In this type of infarct, the right coronary artery is involved, and no reciprocal changes will be seen.

ECG CHANGES PRESENT WHEN THE ANTERIOR, ANTEROLATERAL, ANTEROSEPTAL AND INFERIOR WALLS ARE INVOLVED IN AN INFRACTION

When the anterior wall is affected through an MI, ECG changes include positive R-wave progression and ST segment elevation that can be identified through leads V_1, V_2, V_3, and V_4, with possible reciprocal changes in leads II, III, and aVF. These lead changes indicate that the left coronary artery or the left anterior descending artery is occluded.

When the anterolateral wall is affected, ECG changes can be seen in leads V_1, V_2, V_3, V_4, V_5, and V_6. Reciprocal changes can be seen in leads II, III, and aVF. These changes indicate involvement in the left anterior descending artery or the circumflex artery.

When the anteroseptal wall is affected, ECG changes can be seen in leads V_1, V_2 and V_3, with no reciprocal changes. These ECG changes indicate that the left anterior descending artery may be occluded.

When the inferior wall is affected, ECG changes will be seen in leads II, III and aVF with possible reciprocal change in leads I, aVL, V5 and V6.

CLINICAL MANIFESTATION AND COMPLICATIONS RELATED TO AN ANTERIOR WALL MI

During an anterior wall MI, the patient will show ST segment elevation in leads V_3 and V_4; ST elevations will also be seen in leads V_1 through V_4 if there is septal involvement. These ECG changes indicate an occlusion in the left anterior descending (LAD) coronary artery, as it supplies oxygen to the anterior wall of the heart.

The primary complications related to an anterior wall MI are complete heart blocks and bundle branch blocks, as the LAD supplies oxygenated blood to the bundle branches of the cardiac conduction system. There is also a risk for the development of ventricular septal defect or rupture. Care must be taken with patients who have had an anterior wall infarct as they have an increased risk of left ventricular dysfunction.

CLINICAL MANIFESTATION AND COMPLICATIONS RELATED TO AN INFERIOR WALL MI

During an inferior wall MI, a patient will exhibit ECG changes in leads II, III and aVF. When these types of ECG changes are visualized, it is suspected that the right coronary artery (RCA) is occluded, as it supplies oxygen to the inferior wall of the heart.

Complications of an inferior wall infarct include bradycardia and first and second-degree heart block, as the RCA also provides oxygen to the sinoatrial (SA) and atrioventricular (AV) nodes. An increased level of parasympathetic nervous system activity is seen in patients with inferior wall MI, often resulting in nausea and vomiting. After an inferior wall MI, patients are at risk for papillary muscle rupture.

CLINICAL MANIFESTATIONS RELATED TO A POSTERIOR WALL MI

An infarct of the posterior wall of the heart may not show ECG changes, as no ECG electrodes are placed directly over the posterior wall. However, ST segment depressions may be evident through leads V_1 through V_6, as these leads are reciprocal to the posterior wall. The coronary artery involved in a posterior wall infarction is the posterior descending artery (PDA). In some members of the patient population, the PDA originates from the RCA and may be associated with an inferior wall infarct. Otherwise, the PDA originates from the circumflex artery, and may be associated with a lateral wall infarct.

CLINICAL MANIFESTATION AND COMPLICATIONS RELATED TO A LATERAL WALL MI

A lateral wall MI may be more difficult to diagnose, as ECG changes may be less pronounced. However treatment should be just as aggressive as for an anterior or inferior wall MI because the involved coronary artery (the circumflex) provides oxygen to a large part of the myocardium. During a lateral wall MI, ECG changes may be seen in leads I and aVL.

A patient who is having a lateral wall MI is at particular risk for heart block, as the circumflex artery supplies oxygen for the AV node. Because the circumflex artery also supplies oxygen the papillary muscles, it is important to monitor for a new-onset holosystolic murmur, as this is indicative of papillary muscle dysfunction.

USING TROPONIN AND CREATINE KINASE TO DIAGNOSE STEMI

Troponin is the current biomarker of choice used to diagnose acute MI. Though troponin is found in both skeletal and cardiac muscle tissue, assays have been developed to differentiate between the two. A rise in cardiac troponin is usually seen in the blood 3 to 5 hours after the onset of symptoms, and peak within 10-24 hours. Troponin may remain elevated for 5-14 days after the cardiac event. The exact amount of troponin needed to produce a positive test result is dependent upon the assay used.

Because creatine kinase is found in all skeletal tissue, it is not as accurate as the use of troponin in diagnosing AMI (acute myocardial infarction). Anything that can cause muscle damage, such as a recent fall or heavy exertion, may produce a false positive creatine kinase result. Typically, a CK-MB test is considered to be positive at a level of 0-5 mcg/L. CK-MB levels begin to rise 4-6 hours after the onset of symptoms, and peak after 10-24 hours. However, serum CK-MB levels normalize more quickly (after 2-3 days) and are less specific for damage to the heart muscle than troponin.

USING MYOGLOBIN AND ISCHEMIA-MODIFIED ALBUMIN TO DIAGNOSE ACUTE MI

Myoglobin is a protein released into the bloodstream when damage occurs to muscle tissue. The advantage of a myoglobin test is that is begins to rise 2 to 3 hours after cardiac damage -- earlier than either troponin or creatine kinase. Myoglobin peaks after 6 to 9 hours and normalizes after 12 hours. The disadvantage of a myoglobin test is that it is present in both skeletal and cardiac muscle tissue. Thus, any recent skeletal muscle damage can cause a false positive result.

Ischemia-modified albumin is a relatively new test that is used in conjunction with troponin to quickly diagnose acute myocardial infarction (AMI). The assay is based on the finding that cobalt has an inability to bind effectively to human albumin after an AMI. Ischemia-modified albumin levels rise within 6 to 10 minutes after ischemia, and return to normal levels 6 to 12 hours after the ischemia is corrected.

TREATMENT OF STEMI

EMERGENT TREATMENT OF A STEMI

When the patient is diagnosed with acute MI, steps must be taken to rapidly restore perfusion to the cardiac muscle. Pain relief is provided to the patient, typically in the form of intravenous morphine or fentanyl. The patient is placed on adjunctive oxygen, as well as continuous ECG monitoring to assess cardiac conduction. Aspirin is given for its antiplatelet effect. Nitroglycerine and beta-blockers are given to the patient to reduce cardiac workload, unless patient's heart rate and blood pressure contraindicates receiving the medication.

In the case of STEMI, immediate reperfusion is required. The patient should be prepared for an immediate percutaneous coronary intervention (PCI). The ideal door-to-balloon time (i.e., time from arrival to reperfusion via angioplasty balloon or stent) is 90 minutes or less in order to preserve cardiac muscle and function. In the case of NSTEMI, emergent PCI is not indicated. Intravenous thrombolytic therapy such as streptokinase or tPA should be started within 30 minutes of arrival to the ER to prevent blood clots from further occluding the coronary artery.

OXYGEN ADMINISTRATION

Adjunctive oxygen is provided to patients during an acute MI in an attempt to reduce the extent of the infarct by reducing cardiac workload. It is recommended that oxygen therapy be given to patients during the first six hours after an acute MI, beginning at 2 liters per minute and titrating upward to maintain oxygen saturation greater than 90%. After the initial six hours, adjunctive oxygen is not necessary unless the patient's oxygen saturation remains low.

Care must be taken in patients who have a history of COPD, as some patients rely upon a high level of CO_2 for autonomic respiratory control.

BETA-BLOCKERS

Beta-adrenergic receptor blocking agents or beta-blockers have proven to be effective in treating patients with ST elevation MI. Metoprolol is the beta-blocker of choice. Metoprolol binds to the sympathetic receptors in the heart, decreasing the effect of adrenaline. This results in a decrease in heart rate, cardiac output, and blood pressure, which in turn reduces the oxygen demand of the heart. It is administered as an IV push, at a rate of 5 mg over 5 minutes.

Because beta-blockers work on the $beta_1$ receptors (thereby lowering heart rate and blood pressure), it is contraindicated in patients with a heart rate of less than 60 bpm or where systolic blood pressure is less than 95 mmHg. It is also contraindicated in patients who are in second or third degree heart block, as it may cause asystole. Beta-blockers also have a constricting effect on the bronchioles, thus beta-blockers should not be given to patients with a known history of asthma.

MORPHINE SULFATE

Morphine is given to patients during an acute MI for a number of reasons. It is given as an analgesic, and it helps to relieve anxiety secondary to severe chest pain. Morphine also helps to reduce cardiac preload (ventricular distention), resulting in a decreased cardiac workload.

The typical initial dose of Morphine is 2 to 4 mg given intravenously. Afterward, 2 to 8 mg can be given as an "IV push" every five minutes until the desired effect is achieved.

Care must be taken while administering morphine, as it can act as a respiratory depressant.

ASPIRIN

Aspirin is given to patients during an acute myocardial infarction to help improve the chance of survival. It inhibits platelet aggregation associated with thrombus, and thereby contributes to cardiac muscle perfusion. An adult dosage of 325 mg is typically given orally. Aspirin is considered to be more effective when the patient chews the aspirin tablet rather than swallowing it whole, as this facilitates more rapid medication absorption. It is contraindicated in patients with aspirin allergies.

After discharge, patients should be encouraged to continue taking 325 mg of aspirin daily to help reduce risk of reocclusion. The patient should be monitored, as there is an increased risk for bleeding when taking aspirin.

NITROGLYCERINE

Nitroglycerine is prescribed to patients to help decrease cardiac workload and oxygen demand. It causes vasodilation by stimulating the release of nitric acid from the endothelium. Vasodilation causes a decrease in cardiac afterload (ejection resistance), reducing the amount of force necessary to push blood into the arteries. Venous return is also decreased, as there is an increase in venous capacity. This results in a lower stroke volume and cardiac output.

When the patient is experiencing chest pain, nitroglycerine is the first treatment option, unless contraindicated due to decreased blood pressure. It is initially given sublingually, with one tab placed under the tongue every 5 minutes for three consecutive doses. If the chest pain is not relieved, intravenous nitroglycerine would be next considered, provided the patient's blood pressure remains stable. The initial IV dosage is 10mcg/min. The dose is titrated upward by

10mcg/min every 10 minutes until the chest pain is relieved, provided the patient's blood pressure remains stable.

DISCHARGE PLANNING FOR A PATIENT FOLLOWING STEMI

A patient who has had an acute myocardial infarction (AMI) may be prepared for discharge in a number of ways. Cardiac function is evaluated using a stress test and a blood-flow imaging exam. A 2D echocardiogram may be used to assess valve patency and the cardiac ejection fraction. An implantable cardiac defibrillator (ICD) may be placed for any patient with an ejection fraction less than 40%. A second cardiac catheterization may be done to evaluate persistent chest pain.

Unless contraindicated, a number of medications are started or continued to provide secondary MI prevention. These include beta-blockers and ACE inhibitors (inhibitors of Angiotensin-Converting Enzyme) to lower cardiac workload and prevent reinfarction, statins to minimize further atherosclerotic buildup, and aspirin for its antiplatelet effect. If a patient had an intravascular stent placed, Plavix (clopidogrel) is typically prescribed to prevent reocclusion of the stent.

Cardiac rehabilitation is provided both in-hospital and after discharge. The purpose of this is to identify and manage risk factors, including lifestyle changes such as exercise and diet control.

TREATMENT FOR A PATIENT DIAGNOSED WITH NSTEMI

When a patient presents with chest pain, an ECG should be performed immediately to ensure that there are no ST elevations indicative of a more serious myocardial infarction. The patient will typically be treated with oxygen, aspirin, nitroglycerine, and morphine to decrease cardiac workload and relieve the chest pain.

Continuous ECG monitoring should be performed, and any changes reported to the physician. Investigate and treat any worsening of chest pain. Cardiac enzymes should also be drawn to assess cardiac tissue damage. Repeat testing of appropriate cardiac enzymes may be conducted to monitor any elevation in levels indicative of further extension of the MI, or to confirm that the initial cardiac event is subsiding. Prior to discharge, the patient will receive teaching regarding medical management and lifestyle changes after a NSTEMI.

THROMBOLYTIC THERAPIES FOR NSTEMI

In the case of NSTEMI, thrombolytic therapy is recommended to prevent further occlusion of the coronary artery. The patient is prescribed one of the following four thrombolytics: streptokinase, anisoylated plasminogen streptokinase activator complex (APSAC), tissue plasminogen activator (tPA) and Tenecteplase. A heparin drip is then started six hours after the completion of the thrombolytic therapy, when the patient's aPTT (activated partial thromboplastin time) has reached a level of 70 seconds (i.e., a target window of 50-70 seconds).

The dosage of a streptokinase drip is 1.5 million units, given over a period of 60 minutes. APSAC (anisoylated plasminogen streptokinase activator complex) is given as a 30mg bolus over 5 minutes. The thrombolytic agent tPA is given as a 15mg bolus, followed by a drip rate of 0.75mg/kg, until up to 50mg has infused. The rate is then decreased to 0.5mg/kg up to 35 mg. Tenecteplase is given as an IV push; dosing is dependent upon the weight of the patient, with 30-50mg usually given intravenously over 5 seconds.

During the course of thrombolytic therapy, it is important to monitor the patient for bleeding, using coagulation studies such as PT/PTT and INR. The patient should also be monitored for signs of bloody urine or stool, bleeding from the gums and nosebleeds, as this is a sign of too much anticoagulation.

USING PLAVIX IN THE TREATMENT OF NSTEMI

Plavix (*Clopidogrel bisulfate*) is prescribed to a patient after a NSTEMI, as it works to prevent platelet aggregation and consequent further occlusion of any narrowed coronary arteries. Plavix should be started immediately after the onset of the ischemic event, and continued for at least one month if there are no plans to perform an intervention on the patient. Plavix should be held for seven days if the patient plans to undergo CABG (coronary artery bypass grafting.

The typical dose of Plavix is 300mg given orally to establish a therapeutic level. Afterward, 75mg should be taken by mouth every day until discontinued by the physician. Plavix therapy may require closer monitoring or be contraindicated in cases of liver disease, digestive tract bleeding (i.e., active stomach ulcers, etc.), bleeding in the tissues of the eyes, or in or around the brain, etc. Synergistic effects with other drugs may occur (i.e., the anticoagulant effects of aspirin become more pronounced when taking Plavix).

STABLE ANGINA VS. UNSTABLE ANGINA

Angina is chest pain caused by ischemic damage to myocardial tissue. Atherosclerotic plaque causes a narrowing of the coronary arteries, slowing the flow of oxygenated blood to cardiac cells. Lack of oxygen causes cellular damage, which in turn causes chest pain. In the case of stable angina, the pain begins gradually and gains intensity before dissipating. The chest pain is associated with periods of activity, tachycardia, elevated blood pressure, and with the presence of sympathomimetic drugs. Administration of nitrates usually relieves the pain.

In the case of unstable angina, the chest pain occurs while the patient is at rest. The pain lasts longer than 10 minutes, and it does not respond to the administration nitroglycerine.

Dysrhythmias

NORMAL SINUS RHYTHM

Sinus rhythm is the most common ECG rhythm seen in patients with no cardiac history. The term refers to cardiac contractions that properly originate in the sino-atrial node. In sinus rhythm, the heartbeat is initiated in the sinoatrial (SA) node at a rate between 60 to 100 beats per minutes. The beats occur at regular intervals, and are composed of one P wave, one QRS complex, and one T wave. The P wave starts the cardiac contraction cycle; it indicates atrial systole or depolarization.

The QRS complex occurs after the P wave, and represents ventricular depolarization. It is measured from the first negative deflection (Q wave) through the positive deflection (R wave) to the end of the negative deflection (S wave).

The area from the end of the S wave to the end of the T wave represents ventricular repolarization and relaxation. It is usually measured as part of the QT complex, the area beginning with the Q wave and ending with the T wave.

MEASURING SINUS RHYTHM

The PR interval is measured from the first positive deflection of the isoelectric baseline (the P wave) to the beginning of the QRS complex. The typical duration of the PR interval is 0.12 to 0.20 seconds.

The QRS complex is measured from the first negative deflection from the isoelectric baseline (the Q wave), through the positive deflection (R wave), and ends when the final negative deflection (S wave) returns to baseline. The normal duration of a QRS complex is 0.06 to 0.10 seconds.

The QT interval is measured from the Q wave to the end of the T wave, when the final positive deflection returns to the isoelectric baseline. The normal duration of the QT interval is between 0.36 and 0.44 seconds.

NURSING IMPLICATIONS WHEN MONITORING DYSRHYTHMIAS

When the patient undergoes a cardiac rhythm change, it is important to obtain an ECG and notify the physician of any significant changes. Any heart rate slower than 50 beats per minute or faster than 140 beats per minute may cause a decrease in perfusion, secondary to decreased cardiac output. In these instances, the patient's blood pressure and radial pulse should be closely monitored for hypotension as evidenced by "threadiness."

The patient should also be assessed for chest pain or neurological changes, which may indicate lack of perfusion to the cardiac muscle and brain, respectively. If the patient's skin becomes cool and pale, it indicates lack of peripheral blood flow.

NURSING IMPLICATIONS FOR SINUS BRADYCARDIA

When a patient's heart rate drops below 50-60 beats per minute, it is called sinus bradycardia. If a patient experiences sinus bradycardia, monitor for clinical signs and symptoms of decreased cardiac output, such as neurological changes or chest pain. Proper assessment is important, as bradycardia may be normal for athletes and some patients who are sleeping.

If the patient becomes symptomatic with bradycardia, administer adjunctive oxygen and prepare to begin transcutaneous pacing. Closely monitor blood pressure while the patient's heart rate is low. Atropine may be given intravenously to help elevate the heart rate while transcutaneous pacing is pending.

Bradycardia can be caused by electrolyte imbalance, drug toxicity, excess vagal tone, inferior wall MI, hypoglycemia, increased intracranial pressure, and sick sinus syndrome. The underlying cause for bradycardia should be discovered and corrected.

WOLFF-PARKINSON-WHITE SYNDROME

Wolff-Parkinson-White Syndrome (WPW) occurs when the patient has an extra electrical conduction pathway through the heart. This path, called an accessory pathway, may allow contractile signals to move too quickly through the cardiac conduction system, arriving at the ventricles too soon. Some patients with accessory pathways may never experience complications secondary to WPW syndrome. However, when preexcitation or conduction down the accessory path occurs, it can result in tachycardia with resultant signs of hypoperfusion.

A patient who is symptomatic with WPW syndrome is treated with antiarrhythmics such as Adenocard or procainamide, to decrease excitability within the cardiac tissue and restore primary pacemaker functions to the SA and AV nodes. Close cardiac monitoring is indicated, and oxygen should be administered as needed.

FIRST DEGREE HEART BLOCK

A first-degree atrioventricular (AV) block occurs when there is a conduction delay between the sinoatrial node and the ventricles. The conduction delay most commonly takes place in the AV node, but delays can take place intra-atrially or in the His-Purkinje relay system as well. A first-degree block is characterized by a prolonged PR interval, >0.20 seconds on an ECG.

Patients presenting with a first-degree block generally show no symptoms. However, a first-degree block should be closely monitored, as it can progress to a more serious heart block.

It should be noted that patients who are currently taking calcium channel blockers, beta-blockers, or digoxin may have a prolonged PR interval as these medications slow conduction through the AV node.

TYPE I SECOND-DEGREE BLOCK

A Type I second-degree block (or Mobitz Type I or Wenckebach AV block) occurs when the PR interval gradually lengthens until the P wave fails to conduct to the AV node, resulting in a dropped QRS complex.

A patient with a Type I second-degree block is typically asymptomatic. However, if the conduction block is significant enough to cause decreased cardiac output, the patient might present with light-headedness, syncope, or palpitations. If the patient is symptomatic, a permanent pacemaker may be considered. The patient should be closely monitored as a Type I second degree block may progress to a more serious heart block.

Type I second-degree blocks are most commonly seen in patients who have recently had an inferior wall MI or who have excess vagal tone. If a patient is taking calcium channel blockers, beta-blockers, digoxin, or amiodarone, they may develop a Type I second-degree block.

TYPE II SECOND-DEGREE BLOCK

A Type II second-degree block (also called a Mobitz Type II block) occurs when conduction between the SA node and the AV node is blocked without warning, resulting in a randomly dropped QRS complex. This is visualized on an ECG by a regular R-R interval preceding a P wave with no QRS complex.

If QRS complexes are dropped frequently, the patient may begin showing symptoms of low cardiac output, such as syncope, clammy skin, chest pain, or altered mental status. If the patient is symptomatic while in Mobitz type II, temporary pacing should be considered. Even if asymptomatic, a patient in this type of block must be closely monitored as it may progress to third degree heart block.

THIRD DEGREE HEART BLOCK

Third degree or complete heart block occurs when there is no conduction between the SA and the AV nodes. Both P waves and QRS complexes are present. The P to P intervals are regular, as are the QRS to QRS intervals, but there is no correlation between the P waves and the QRS complexes. Consequently, P waves may be seen to "march through" or "hide" in the QRS complexes or T waves. Because there is no correlation between the SA node and the AV node, the patient's ventricular rate drops to 20 to 40 beats per minute. The slow rhythm causes syncope, chest pain, lightheadedness, and/or altered mental status.

When a patient presents with third degree heart block, temporary pacing should be considered. A permanent pacemaker will be required if the complete heart block continues to occur.

CAUSES OF HEART BLOCKS

There are multiple potential causes of the various heart blocks. Certain medications, particularly those prescribed for tachyarrhythmias, can cause heart blocks as they slow conduction through the heart. These can include amiodarone, calcium channel blockers, beta-blockers, and digoxin. If possible, when a block occurs, it is recommended that any related medication be discontinued to avoid the progression of a minor block to a more serious block.

Coronary artery disease and acute myocardial infarction can cause a heart block as a result of cardiac tissue damage. Rheumatic fever and hyperkalemia are other potential causes of heart block.

TREATMENT GOALS FOR A HEART BLOCK

Treatment is not required if a patient is asymptomatic while in a minor heart block. If possible, treatment of the underlying cause is necessary to prevent progression to a more serious block. If the patient becomes bradycardic with symptoms or hypoperfusion, intravenous atropine may be required.

In the case of complete heart block, close ECG monitoring is essential. If the patient becomes symptomatic as a result of the bradycardia, immediate transcutaneous pacing may be necessary. Elevating the heart rate, either with pacing or intravenous atropine, can relieve the signs of hypoperfusion. If a third-degree block is chronic, then permanent pacing may be required.

PREMATURE VENTRICULAR CONTRACTIONS

Premature ventricular contractions (PVC's) are early QRS complexes caused by the premature stimulation of the ventricles. This errant stimulation may be caused by irritable ventricular pacemaker cells. A PVC after every other beat is called bigeminy. A PVC after every second heartbeat is referred to as trigeminy. PVCs cause no problems for a person with an otherwise healthy heart. However, care should be taken with a person with a history of cardiac problems as PVC's can trigger ventricular tachycardia.

PVC's can be caused by medications such as cardiac glycosides or sympathomimetic agents, anxiety, caffeine, hypoxia, or myocardial ischemia. Electrolyte imbalances such as hypokalemia and hypocalcemia can also cause PVC's. Patients experiencing PVC's may have an irregular pulse. If the PVC's occur frequently enough, the patient may have signs and symptoms of hypoperfusion.

TREATMENT PLAN FOR PVC'S

If the patient starts having symptoms of hypoperfusion combined with multiple PVC's (premature ventricular contractions), it will be necessary to provide a medical response. The primary goal of managing PVC's is to correct the underlying cause of the condition. Intravenous amiodarone can be administered to treat the irritable cardiac cells. Intravenous atropine should be considered for symptomatic bradycardia. The underlying cause of the PVC's, however, must still be found and treated.

Nursing implications include continuous ECG monitoring, and administering oxygen and antiarrhythmics. Close monitoring of the patient for signs of hypoperfusion is important. If the PVC's initiate ventricular tachycardia, prompt administration of CPR and defibrillation will be required.

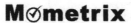

CAUSES AND EVIDENCE FOR JUNCTIONAL RHYTHMS

Junctional rhythms occur when the SA node fails to generate an impulse. The AV node then acts as a backup pacemaker a period of SA node failure. This is typically seen during sinus bradycardia or with second- or third-degree heart block.

However, when the AV node functions as the primary pacemaker of the heart, the heart rate is considerably slower than when the SA node functions as the primary pacemaker. A junctional rhythm produces a narrow QRS complex on ECG. An accelerated junctional rhythm may also occur (rate >60), and will also appear as a narrowed complex rhythm on ECG. The QRS complexes are uniform in shape, and a retrograde P wave activation may or may not be present. During a junctional rhythm, the ventricular rate usually remains approximately 20 to 60 beats per minute. Some patients are unable to tolerate this decreased rate, and may show signs and symptoms of hypoperfusion, such as syncope, decreased level of consciousness, or hypotension.

ASYSTOLE

In cases of asystole, no electrical activity can be seen within the heart. It is characterized on an ECG by a flat line. The patient is unresponsive and no pulse can be felt. It is caused by failed cardiac conduction or prolonged periods of poor oxygenation.

In some cases, pulseless electrical activity (PEA) may be seen on the monitor. This is the result of a complete disconnect between the cardiac conduction system and mechanical activities. This results in a visual electrical conduction pattern on the ECG, but no pulse will be felt.

When asystole occurs, it is important to confirm it via two different leads to ensure that all cardiac leads are actually in place. CPR should be initiated, starting with compressions, using a 30 compressions to 2 breaths ratio until the patient is intubated in which case compressions are continuous and the patient is ventilated at a rate of one breath per 5-6 seconds. Intravenous epinephrine should be administered as soon as possible, 1mg every 3 to 5 minutes. Asystole and PEA are not shockable rhythms, therefore defibrillation is not indicated.

NURSING IMPLICATIONS FOR SINUS ARREST

Sinus arrest occurs when the sinoatrial (SA) node fails to initiate an impulse, resulting in missing PQRST complexes (i.e., "beats"). This is sometimes referred to as "sinus pause" (a term encompassing both sinus arrest and sinus exit block). The patient may present with cool clammy skin or altered mental status, and other symptoms associated with decreased cardiac output.

Sinus arrest may be caused by drug toxicity, ischemia of the SA node, sick sinus syndrome, or excess vagal tone. If the patient is experiencing pauses and is symptomatic, it is important to administer oxygen to decrease cardiac workload. Atropine may be given intravenously. The patient may also need temporary transcutaneous pacing until the underlying cause can be corrected, or a permanent pacer placed if the problem cannot be corrected.

NURSING IMPLICATIONS OF SINUS TACHYCARDIA

Sinus tachycardia presents with a fast sinus rhythm, with heart beats between 100 to 160 beats per minute. At these increased rates, the ventricles have less filling time. As a result, cardiac output decreases. The patient may show symptoms of decreased perfusion, such as mental status changes, or cool and clammy skin. If the patient is symptomatic with sinus tachycardia, it is important to administer oxygen and any prescribed medications, such as beta-blockers or Cardizem.

Sinus tachycardia can be caused by anxiety, pain, exercise, or stimulants such as certain medications, nicotine, or caffeine. It is important to treat the underlying cause of the sinus tachycardia and correct it.

VENTRICULAR TACHYCARDIA

Ventricular tachycardia ("V-tach" or VT) occurs when the patient has multiple PVC's in a row, at a rate of 100 to 250 beats per minute. Because the rate is so quick, the ventricles are unable to fill effectively, resulting in a drop in cardiac output. V-tach is caused by myocardial tissue damage resulting in increased irritability of the cardiac cells. This irritability can be caused by myocardial infarction, cardiomyopathy, or congestive heart failure. Ventricular tachycardia can also be caused by pulmonary embolus, hypokalemia, or hypoxemia. Drug toxicity from epinephrine and digoxin can also cause V-tach.

A patient in ventricular tachycardia will have either no palpable pulse, or one that is only faintly palpable. If the decreased cardiac output is not compensated, the patient will become unresponsive. If the patient loses consciousness, immediate defibrillation and administration of CPR is essential.

TORSADES DE POINTES

The term "torsades de points" is a literal translation from the French phrase "twisting of the points," and it refers to an uncommon variant of V-tach. It is characterized on an ECG by a twisting of the QRS complex into a helical shape around an isoelectric baseline. Because ventricular depolarization occurs at a rapid rate, signs of hypoperfusion will be seen in a patient with torsades. If left untreated, the patient will progress into ventricular fibrillation.

Torsades are preceded by a lengthening QT interval, usually greater than one-half the R-to-R interval. This can occur as a result of electrolyte imbalance such as hypomagnesaemia or hypokalemia, as well as medication therapy or cardiac ischemia. Managing torsades with group IA antidysrhythmic drugs can have dire results, thus a proper diagnosis is essential. Prompt cardioversion is the primary treatment for torsades, as well as intravenous magnesium and correction of the underlying cause of the lengthened QT interval.

NURSING IMPLICATIONS FOR SUPRAVENTRICULAR TACHYCARDIA

Supraventricular tachycardia (SVT) is a rhythm that originates from the sinoatrial (SA) node. The heart beats at a rate between 150-250 beats per minute. As a result of this substantially increased rate, ventricular filling is greatly decreased. The patient may present with altered mental status or cardiac ischemia secondary to decreased perfusion.

SVT is characterized by narrowed QRS complexes, and the P waves are unable to be visualized as they are obscured by the T waves. Causes of SVT include myocardial infarction, valvular disease, hyperthyroidism, cor pulmonale, or digoxin toxicity.

If the patient is asymptomatic with the SVT, encourage the patient to perform vagal maneuvers such as coughing or the Valsalva maneuver. Medications such as calcium channel blockers or Adenocard may be administered to try and return the patient to a normal rhythm. If the patient is symptomatic with the SVT, prepare for emergent cardioversion. If the SVT does not respond to medical management, radiofrequency ablation may be necessary to correct it.

VENTRICULAR FIBRILLATION

Ventricular fibrillation ("V-fib" or VF) usually occurs as a result of cardiac ischemia, secondary to acute MI or untreated ventricular tachycardia. It can also be caused by hypothermia, acid-base imbalances, and hypoxemia. Electrolyte imbalances such as hypokalemia, hyperkalemia or hypercalcemia can also cause V-fib.

V-fib is characterized on an ECG by either coarse or fine fibrillating waves. These waves are a result of rapid and chaotic depolarization of the cardiac cells, causing the heart muscle to quiver rather than contract. A patient in V-fib has no pulse, and quickly becomes unresponsive. In treating V-fib, it is clinically accepted that coarse V-fib is easier to convert to sinus rhythm than fine V-fib. Immediate defibrillation and CPR, as well as correction of the underlying cause are the appropriate treatments for V-fib.

TREATMENT PLAN FOR V-FIB AND V-TACH

If a patient experiences ventricular tachycardia or ventricular fibrillation, immediate action is required. If the patient is conscious and asymptomatic in cases of V-tach, amiodarone or lidocaine should be administered intravenously. If the amiodarone is ineffective, emergent cardioversion will be necessary.

If the patient loses consciousness, the patient should be defibrillated immediately and CPR initiated to continue circulation. Epinephrine or a single dose of vasopressin may be administered. Antiarrhythmics such as amiodarone or lidocaine may also be administered intravenously.

If the V-tach or V-fib is recurrent, an implanted cardioverter-defibrillator (ICD) will be necessary.

ATRIAL FLUTTER AND ATRIAL FIBRILLATION

Atrial fibrillation occurs when multiple irritable areas throughout the atria fire at a rate of up to 350-600 times a minute, causing the atria to quiver with an irregular rhythm, rather than effectively contract to fill the ventricles. Because the AV node is unable relay impulses occurring at such a fast pace, most do not reach the ventricles. Some, however, will penetrate and cause the ventricles to contract with an irregular rhythm. Atrial fibrillation is visualized on an ECG with no PR interval, and a baseline that appears wavy or chaotic.

In atrial flutter, the multiple impulses originate from the same area of the atria, firing at a rate of 250 to 350 times per minute. However, the atrial rhythm is regular as opposed to irregular. The AV node may filter out many of these errant charges to control the ventricular rate, thus it may be regular or irregular. Atrial flutter is characterized by saw-toothed flutter waves on an ECG.

Both atrial fibrillation and atrial flutter need to be monitored, as the increased ventricular rate may lead to decreased perfusion and hypotension.

TREATMENTS AVAILABLE FOR ATRIAL FIBRILLATION AND FLUTTER

Atrial flutter and fibrillation are treated in a number of ways. The type of treatment used is dependent upon the patient's presentation. If the patient is asymptomatic, then a medical management approach is the first step. Medical management of atrial fibrillation/flutter involves the use of beta-blockers, calcium channel blockers, and digitalis to slow the ventricular response. Antiarrhythmic agents such as amiodarone may be given to suppress the irritable atrial cells, allowing the SA node to be the dominant pacemaker. Anticoagulants such as Coumadin or Heparin are also provided to prevent thromboembolic disorders.

If medical management is unsuccessful, the next consideration would be radiofrequency ablation or cardioversion.

COMPLICATIONS RELATED TO ATRIAL FIBRILLATION OR ATRIAL FLUTTER

When a patient is in atrial fibrillation or flutter, they may show signs and symptoms of decreased perfusion. The atria are unable to produce a coordinated contraction, causing less blood to be pushed into the ventricles. Stroke volume is thus affected, leading to a decreased cardiac output.

A patient in atrial flutter or fibrillation is also at risk for thromboembolic disorders such as a stroke or pulmonary embolism. Blood clots may form in the atria as a result of the inadequate strength of the contraction, which may then be expelled into the brain or lungs. Therefore, it is important for patients diagnosed with atrial flutter or fibrillation to be placed on anticoagulants such as Coumadin to prevent a thromboembolic syndrome.

The third potential complication of atrial flutter or fibrillation is rapid ventricular response (RVR). In RVR, the AV node is unable to properly filter the multiple impulses emerging from the atria, resulting in an increased ventricular rate. A patient in atrial fibrillation or flutter with RVR may complain of dizziness, shortness of breath, diaphoresis or chest pain secondary to decreased cardiac output or decreased coronary perfusion.

RATE CONTROL IN ATRIAL FIBRILLATION
BETA-BLOCKERS

Beta-adrenergic receptor blockers or beta-blockers include medications such as Lopressor (Metoprolol), Inderal (Propranolol), or Betapace (Sotalol). They are prescribed for patients in atrial fibrillation or flutter because they prolong the atrial refractory period, slowing the rate of conduction through the SA and AV nodes. They also decrease the destabilizing effects of the sympathetic nervous system by binding to the adrenaline receptors, further preventing an elevated heart rate.

Side effects of beta-blockers include heart block, nausea, constipation, and dizziness. Beta-blockers are contraindicated for patients with a history of asthma as they may cause bronchospasm.

CALCIUM CHANNEL BLOCKERS

Calcium channel blockers include medications such as Cardizem (Diltiazem), Norvasc (Amlodipine), Plendil (Felodipine) or Verapamil (Isoptin). They help control the rate in atrial fibrillation or flutter by inhibiting the calcium channel pump within cardiac cells, prolonging the amount of time it takes for the cell to repolarize. This has a negative chronotropic effect, as depolarization cannot take place until repolarization has been completed.

Side effects of calcium channel blockers include heart block, dizziness, peripheral edema, headache, and constipation. Calcium channel blockers are contraindicated for patients who have a history of sick sinus syndrome or left ventricular dysfunction.

DIGOXIN

Digoxin is also referred to as Digitalis, Lanoxin or Digitek. It is prescribed to patients in atrial fibrillation or flutter because it increases vagal activity, resulting in an increased parasympathetic response within the heart. This slows the firing of the pacemaker cells, decreasing the number of impulses sent to the AV node. An increased parasympathetic response also counteracts the sympathetic nervous system, causing a slower heart rate.

Patients taking digoxin may complain of loss of appetite, palpitations, nausea, dizziness, and/or visual disturbances. Digoxin is contraindicated for patients who have a history of ventricular fibrillation or have a hypersensitivity to the medication.

Because of its narrow therapeutic range, frequent blood tests are required to ensure appropriate dosing.

PHARMACOLOGIC EFFECTS OF ATROPINE AND EPINEPHRINE

Atropine is a competitive antagonist for acetylcholine, the neurotransmitter used by the parasympathetic nervous system. It binds to acetylcholine receptors without activating them, decreasing the effectiveness of the parasympathetic nervous system. This results in an increased rate of firing within the SA node as well as more effective conduction through the AV node. The typical dose of atropine is 0.5 to 1 mg intravenously every 3 to 5 minutes, up to a maximum dosage of 0.04 mg per kilogram.

Epinephrine is the neurotransmitter of the sympathetic nervous system. It works by causing systemic vasoconstriction, which pushes blood from the peripheral vascular system to the heart. It also binds to the cardiac beta-receptors, resulting in increased heart rate and increased cardiac output. The typical dose of epinephrine is 0.5 to 1 mg given intravenously every 3 to 5 minutes. There is no maximum dosage for epinephrine. If administered through an endotracheal tube, the dosage is 2 to 2.5 times the IV dosage.

Heart Failure

Heart failure is defined as the inability of the heart to meet the oxygen requirements of the body. In an adult, heart failure can be precipitated by structural abnormalities such as ventricular septal defect or valvular insufficiency, or by functional abnormalities such as decreased ventricular contractility. It is characterized by complaints of shortness of breath and fatigue.

Heart failure is typically an incurable condition that must be managed properly to avoid an exacerbation of symptoms. Treatment involves medical management and lifestyle changes to compensate for the decreased pumping ability of the heart.

> **Review Video: <u>Congestive Heart Failure</u>**
> Visit mometrix.com/academy and enter code: 924118

CAUSES OF HEART FAILURE

The most common cause of heart failure is loss of contractility secondary to myocardial infarction. Injured cardiac tissue is replaced by scar tissue, which lacks contractility and conductivity. As a result, the ventricle cannot eject an adequate amount of blood.

Heart failure may also be brought on by hypertension. When the cardiac afterload is increased, the left ventricle must work harder to compensate for the increased intravascular pressure. This can lead to ventricular hypertrophy and decreased stroke volume as the thickened ventricular wall decreased the ventricle's blood volume capacity.

Valve failure can also lead to heart failure. If valvular insufficiency is present, the left ventricle must work harder to sustain the forward movement of blood. This can lead to hypertrophy and decreased cardiac output.

Heart failure can also be caused by diabetes, congenital birth defects, and tachycardia secondary to tachyarrhythmias and anemia.

SIGNS AND SYMPTOMS OF HEART FAILURE

The signs and symptoms of heart failure are varied, but typically stem from increased cardiac workload and decreased oxygen saturation. The patient may have complaints of fatigue, dyspnea, or increased anxiety secondary to feelings of suffocation. They may be pale, cyanotic, or diaphoretic. The patient may present with pulmonary crackles on auscultation and a persistent cough as a result of pulmonary congestion. An S3 gallop may be noted when assessing heart tones. Because the body is compensating for decreased cardiac output by the reabsorption of water and sodium, the patient will show signs of fluid overload, such as peripheral edema, jugular venous distension, hepatojugular reflex, and ascites.

DIAGNOSIS OF HEART FAILURE

A patient who presents with signs and symptoms of heart failure will typically be diagnosed based upon their relevant medical history. A 2D echocardiograph may be performed to assess cardiac function and estimate the patient's ejection fraction. A chest X-ray may be done to assess fluid buildup within the lungs.

A blood test to assess levels of B-type natriuretic peptide (BNP) should be obtained to confirm the presence of heart failure. Elevated BNP levels occur when ventricular pressure is high, and ventricular expansion increases. BNP is released into the bloodstream in response to ventricular expansion. BNP levels greater than 100 pg/ml (picograms per milliliter) is indicative of heart failure.

CAUSES AND RISKS FOR ACUTE HEART FAILURE

Acute heart failure can occur as sudden onset, with the body attempting to compensate for circulatory malfunction by protecting blood flow to vital organs. There is an increase in the contractibility of the myocardium but peripheral vasoconstriction. Fluid and sodium are retained to control hypotension. However, the increased contractibility and heart rate increase the need for oxygen beyond that available, leading to physiologic responses that result in tissue necrosis, cardiotoxicity, ischemia, pulmonary edema, and organ failure:

- **Capillary hypertension** decreases oncotic pressure and results in vasodilation and increased loss of fluid from the plasma to the interstitial fluid, resulting in pulmonary edema.
- **Capillary hypotension** results in increased oncotic pressure and pulls fluid back into the plasma, a result of shock.

Acute heart failure may be precipitated by pulmonary embolism, infection, severe arrhythmia, MI, anaphylaxis, and infection. Those with pre-existing cardiac and coronary artery disease, hypertension, diabetes, and renal disease are at increased risk as well as those with excessive use of alcohol and recreational drug use (such as cocaine).

CARDIAC IMPLICATIONS OF ACUTE HEART FAILURE

Acute heart failure (AHF) is a new onset of symptoms or an exacerbation of pre-existing heart failure. Symptoms include cough and dyspnea from pulmonary edema (usually from accumulation of fluids rather than fluid overload). Peripheral edema is less common. A hypertensive crisis may occur. Multiple body systems may be impacted by fluid accumulation:

Cardiovascular implications: JVD noted and positive hepatojugular reflux. Third heart sound evident. Natriuretic peptides increase with heart failure:

Test	Normal	Findings with AHF
BNP	<100 pg/mL or ng/L.	>100 pg/mL or ng/L. Also increased with MI, myocarditis, ventricular dysfunction, and left ventricular hypertrophy.
ProBNP (N-terminal)	0-75 years: <125 pg/mL or ng/L >75 years: <449 pg/mL or ng/mL	>450 pg/mL or ng/L if under age 50 >900 pg/mL or ng/L if ≥ age 50.
ECG	Findings include prolonged QRS, junctional rhythm, elevated ST segment, and prolonged QTC interval. Various arrhythmias may be evident.	

GI AND HEPATIC SYSTEM INDICATIONS OF ACUTE HEART FAILURE

Acute heart failure (AHF) may impact multiple systems in addition to cardiac:

- **Gastrointestinal**: Patients may have nausea, vomiting, abdominal discomfort, and ascites.
- **Hepatic**: The liver may become congested and tender. Hepatomegaly may be noted on palpation and signs of jaundice may be evident.

Test	Normal	Findings with AHF
AST (SGOT)	Male 20-49: 20-40 U/L or 0.34-0.68 micro kat/L	Increases with liver cell damage resulting from hypoperfusion of the liver.
	Male >50: 10-35 U/L or 0.17-0.6 micro kat/L	
	Female 20-45: 15-30 U/L or 0.26-0.51 micro kat/L	
	Female >45: 10-35 U/L or 0.17-0.6 micro kat/L	
ALT (SGPT)	Male 13-60: 10-40 U/L	Increases with liver cell damage resulting from hypoperfusion of the liver.
	Male >60:13-40 U/L	
	Female 13-60:7-35 U/L	
	Female >60: 10-28 U/L	

RENAL AND PULMONARY SYSTEM INDICATIONS OF ACUTE HEART FAILURE

Acute heart failure (AHF) may impact multiple systems in addition to cardiac, GI, and hepatic:

- **Renal**: Urinary output decreases. Laboratory tests:

Test	Normal	Findings with AHF
Serum creatinine	Male: 0.61-1.21 mg/dL or 54-107 mmol/L	Increased, associated with fluid retention and decreased urine output.
	Female: 0.51-1.11 mg/dL or 45-98 mmol/L	
Serum sodium	135-145 mEq/L or mmol/L	Decreased because of reduced cardiac capacity from impaired blood flow to kidneys.

- **Pulmonary**: Patients exhibit dyspnea, orthopnea and PND, tachypnea, wheezing and rales on auscultation.

Test	Findings with AHF
Chest x-ray	Evidence of pleural effusion and pulmonary (interstitial and alveolar) edema.
Ultrasound	B lines indicating presence of interstitial edema.

SYSTOLIC AND DIASTOLIC DYSFUNCTION

Systolic dysfunction occurs when the left ventricle is unable to pump enough blood to meet the oxygen demands of the body. It is typically seen in patients with an ejection fraction less than 50%.

Diastolic dysfunction occurs when the left ventricle is unable to fill properly during diastole. It typically results from decreased compliance in the ventricle secondary to scar tissue or by decreased filling time secondary to conduction abnormalities.

Both systolic and diastolic dysfunction will result in decreased cardiac output secondary to decreased stroke volume. To compensate, the patient may develop an elevated heart rate. Contractility may increase as well, putting the patient at risk for loss of cardiac tone as the muscle becomes overstretched.

LEFT VENTRICULAR DYSFUNCTION

Left ventricular dysfunction is often caused by scar tissue formation on the left ventricle, usually after an acute MI, which causes a decrease in conductivity and elasticity. Heart failure occurs because the left ventricle fails to effectively supply oxygenated blood to the body. Early signs of heart failure include an elevated heart rate coupled with a decrease in blood pressure. The patient may experience poor tolerance to activity. Extra heart tones, particularly an S_3, will be noted on auscultation. Decreased urinary output, with elevated BUN and Creatinine, may occur secondary to decreased blood flow to the kidneys.

Left ventricular dysfunction is managed with lifestyle changes and medication. The patient should be instructed to moderate their physical activity and restrict their sodium and fluid intake. ACE inhibitors and beta-blockers are prescribed to decrease cardiac workload. Diuretics are prescribed to prevent fluid overload. Positive inotropes such as digoxin are prescribed to increase contractility.

HEART FAILURE TREATMENT
ACE INHIBITORS

Angiotensin Converting Enzyme (ACE) inhibitors such as Enalapril (Vasotec), Captopril (Capoten), and Lisinopril (Prinivil) are the first medications considered when treating heart failure. Their pharmacological effect is to prevent the conversion of Angiotensin I to Angiotensin II. Angiotensin II is responsible for the reabsorption of water and sodium, and also acts as a vasoconstrictor. By inhibiting the production of Angiotensin II, the patient experiences fewer fluid-overload symptoms and a consequent decrease in morbidity.

Because ACE inhibitors cause vasodilation, it is important to closely monitor the patient's blood pressure. Renal function should also be carefully monitored, as ACE inhibitors can be nephrotoxic.

ARB'S

Angiotensin II Receptor Blockers (ARB's) such as Losartan (Cozaar) or Valsartan (Diovan) are often prescribed in conjunction with ACE inhibitors in heart failure patients. Treatment with ACE inhibitors may be augmented with ARB's because ACE inhibitors alone may not completely prevent the formation of Angiotensin II. ARB's are typically prescribed to prevent the binding of any additional Angiotensin II to Angiotensin receptors. As a result, vasoconstriction and fluid and sodium retention is reduced.

When initiating ARB therapy, the patient's blood pressure must be closely monitored. The dosage to the prescribed medication must be carefully titrated to ensure the patient does not become hypotensive. ARB's may also cause nausea, vomiting, and headaches.

BETA-BLOCKERS

Beta-blockers have only recently been approved in the treatment of heart failure (Coreg (carvedilol) was first approved for this purpose in 2006). However, they have proven to be effective in decreasing morbidity and mortality. Beta-blockers are prescribed to decrease the levels of systemic catecholamines such as dopamine, epinephrine, and norepinephrine. The decrease causes vasodilation and decreased cardiac workload. Carvedilol, Bisoprolol, and Metoprolol Succinate are currently the beta-blockers of choice.

Because beta-blockers can cause hypotension, it is important to carefully monitor the patient's blood pressure before and after medication administration. It is also important to monitor for the presence of adventitious (abnormal) breath sounds such as wheezes in the lungs, as beta-blockers can cause bronchospasm.

DIGOXIN

Digoxin (Lanoxin) is prescribed to patients with heart failure to increase the contractility of cardiac muscle. Increased contractility encourages forward blood flow, decreasing pulmonary congestion. Digoxin also decreases cardiac workload by functioning as a negative chronotrope.

Frequent blood tests must be done to monitor the patient's digoxin level, as patients who maintain therapeutic levels of digoxin show fewer physical symptoms related to heart failure. The patient may complain of nausea, vomiting, or dizziness if their digoxin level is too high. The patient may also experience bradycardia as a result of the medication's negative chronotropic effect.

DIURETICS

Patients in heart failure routinely suffer from fluid overload. Diuretics are prescribed to remove excess fluid and sodium from the body. Diuretics include medications such as Furosemide (Lasix),

Hydrochlorothiazide (HydroDIURIL), and Spironolactone (Aldactone). Diuretics work by inducing the kidney to remove additional fluid and sodium, which are then excreted as urine. Because patients can develop a tolerance to a diuretic, is important to start with the minimum effective dosage and titrate upward only as necessary.

It is imperative that the patient's electrolyte balance be closely monitored, as other electrolytes can also be excreted out with the intended fluid and sodium. Hypokalemia is the most common electrolyte imbalance seen in patients taking diuretics. However, the patient can also experience depleted magnesium, thiamine, and calcium.

Review Video: <u>Diuretics</u>
Visit mometrix.com/academy and enter code: 373276

NESIRITIDE

Nesiritide (Natrecor) is a synthetic BNP (B-type natriuretic peptide) given to help alleviate symptoms of heart failure. It is given as an intravenous infusion, started after an initial weight-based bolus. Nesiritide imitates the effect of BNP, encouraging diuresis and causing an increased excretion of sodium. This results in a decrease in central venous pressure, as well as a decrease in systemic vascular resistance.

Because Nesiritide causes natriuresis (sodium excretion) and enhances diuresis as a result, it is particularly important to monitor the patient for hypotension while they are receiving the infusion. It is also important to monitor electrolyte levels to ensure that the patient maintains therapeutic levels of potassium, magnesium, and calcium.

TEACHING FOR PATIENTS DIAGNOSED WITH HEART FAILURE

Patient education after a diagnosis of heart failure is important to encourage compliance with the course of treatment. It is important that the patient understand the reasoning behind difficult lifestyle changes involved in ensuring a favorable prognosis.

Fluid and sodium restriction helps to maintain fluid balance and allow the medications to work at an optimum level. A patient in heart failure should take in less than 2gm of sodium daily, and limit fluids to 1000 to 1500 ml a day.

Close weight monitoring is also important. A weight gain of 2 to 4 pounds in 1 to 2 days should be reported to their physician, as it may be an indication of fluid retention.

Other Cardiac Issues and Complications

CARDIAC TAMPONADE

The pericardial sac is the protective lining around the heart. It consists of a fibrous sac and layer of lubricating fluid that allows the heart to move smoothly within the sac. In cardiac tamponade, fluid accumulates in the pericardial sac. This results in increased pressure on the heart, and limits the ability of the atria and ventricles to refill. It thereby decreases stroke volume, often leading to shock and death.

The patient population most at risk for cardiac tamponade would be those with a previous diagnosis of cancer, particularly those with lung or breast cancer, or lymphoma or leukemia. Those patients, especially when undergoing radiation or taking antineoplastic agents, are most at risk.

Patients with hypothyroidism are also at risk for developing cardiac tamponade. Patients who have recently experienced chest trauma should also be closely monitored for cardiac tamponade. Finally, cardiac tamponade may occur as a complication of coronary artery bypass grafting (CABG), central venous catheter or pacemaker insertion, or cardiac catheterization.

TESTS USED TO DIAGNOSE CARDIAC TAMPONADE

A 2D echo is considered the best way to diagnose cardiac tamponade. It can show decreased blood flow through the valves, collapse of the right ventricular wall during diastole, or compression of the right atrium. A chest radiograph may show an enlarged pericardial sac. A 12 lead ECG will show sinus tachycardia, ST segment elevations or low voltage QRS complexes. Pulsus paradoxus will be noted when using pulse oximetry and blood pressure monitoring. A Swan-Ganz catheter can be placed to assess PA and CVP pressures.

A number of blood tests can be drawn to ascertain the cause of the cardiac tamponade. These include HIV serology, creatine kinase and troponin, coagulation profile, complete blood count and renal profile.

SIGNS AND SYMPTOMS OF CARDIAC TAMPONADE

The classic signs of cardiac tamponade are hypotension, jugular venous distension (from decreased of venous return), and muffled heart sounds from fluid buildup in the pericardial sac. These signs are referred to as "Beck's triad." The patient may also experience pulsus paradoxus, a condition in which the patient's blood pressure decreases during inspiration. The patient may also have nausea, vomiting, tachycardia, shortness of breath, abdominal distension, and a decreased level of consciousness.

During cardiac tamponade, the patient will experience increased CVP and PA pressures. The patient will also have decreased stroke volume and cardiac output.

TREATMENT OF CARDIAC TAMPONADE

The primary goal of treatment for cardiac tamponade is to decrease cardiac workload, maintain an appropriate cardiac output, and removal of the excess fluid from within the pericardial sac. The patient should be placed on adjunctive oxygen to increase oxygen perfusion. Fluid volume should be maintained using packed red blood cells, plasma, and crystalloid solutions. Positive inotropes, such as dobutamine or dopamine can be used to increase cardiac output without increasing systemic vascular resistance.

A pericardiocentesis will be done to remove excess fluid from the pericardial sac. The procedure is performed during an echocardiogram by which to guide the needle. The needle is inserted into the chest cavity beneath the xiphoid process, and pierces the pericardial sac. The extra fluid is then slowly drawn out of the pericardial sac using a syringe. Often, the needle can then be replaced with a drainage catheter to remove any additional fluid that may accumulate.

NURSE'S ROLE IN PERICARDIOCENTESIS

The nurse's role in pericardiocentesis includes providing education to the patient regarding the procedure. The nurse also assists by ensuring the appropriate supplies are at hand during the procedure. Prior to the start of the pericardiocentesis, the patient should be helped into a semi-Fowler's position. Sedation is then administered as prescribed, and the patient's airway is monitored and protected. During the procedure, the nurse should monitor the patient's oxygen status, vital signs, and cardiac rate and rhythm. The drainage from the pericardial sac should be collected and saved, as it is usually sent for cytology and pathology testing. The volume of fluid loss through the procedure will also need to be noted.

PERICARDIAL WINDOW

A pericardial window is an operation done while the patient is under general anesthesia. A small incision is made below the sternum to gain access to the pericardial sac. A piece of the pericardial sac is then removed and a drain is placed in the opening. This helps in removal of excess fluid around the heart, and also prevents the subsequent accumulation of additional fluid.

The patient should be carefully monitored after the surgery for signs and symptoms of bleeding, infection, or pleural effusion. The patient should be kept on continuous ECG monitoring and pulse oximetry until stable. Prophylactic antibiotic therapy should be considered.

BLUNT CARDIAC TRAUMA

Blunt cardiac trauma, resulting in a cardiac contusion, typically occurs after a high velocity blow to the chest. The most common cause of blunt cardiac trauma is motor vehicle accidents. Symptoms of blunt cardiac trauma are varied, ranging in severity from mild chest pain to cardiogenic shock. The most common symptom of blunt cardiac trauma is tachycardia.

The patient should be placed on adjunctive oxygen and continuous ECG monitoring. Cardiac biomarkers can be drawn to assess the extent of cardiac tissue damage, and a complete blood count can be done to assess for bleeding. A 2D echocardiograph should be considered, to assess for pericardial effusions. Treatment is based upon the severity of the trauma.

CARDIOGENIC SHOCK

In cardiogenic shock, the heart fails to pump enough blood to provide adequate oxygen to the body. It is characterized by hypotension and altered mental status secondary to decreased cerebral circulation. The patient will also have oliguria (urinary output less than 30ml per hour) as a result of decreased blood flow to the kidneys. During cardiogenic shock, the patient may also experience tachypnea or tachycardia. Their extremities may be cool. Signs of fluid overload such as jugular venous distension and pulmonary edema may be noted. Cardiogenic shock is a fatal condition if it is not treated quickly.

CAUSES OF CARDIOGENIC SHOCK

The primary cause of cardiogenic shock is acute myocardial infarction. The patient is at greatest risk following an anterior wall MI. Sudden loss in cardiac muscle integrity, such as in papillary muscle rupture or ventricular septal rupture, can also induce cardiogenic shock.

Inflammatory conditions such as myocarditis or endocarditis may lead to cardiogenic shock. The patient is also at risk following a long period in a tachyarrhythmia.

Care should be taken with medications that cause hypotension, as these too can cause cardiogenic shock. The medications primarily suspected include ACE inhibitors, beta-blockers and calcium channel blockers.

DIAGNOSIS OF CARDIOGENIC SHOCK

An ECG can be done to show any ST segment elevations that may indicate the presence of an acute myocardial infarction. A 2D echo is helpful in showing structural and functional abnormalities of the heart. It can also help diagnose potential causes such as papillary muscle rupture or ventricular septal rupture. Further, it can show decreased ventricular wall motion and be used estimate the cardiac ejection fraction, as well, to confirm low cardiac output. A portable chest X-ray can be done to diagnose pulmonary edema or cardiomegaly.

Arterial blood gases can be drawn to determine if the body is being properly oxygenated. Renal function tests and liver function tests may be done to assess overall organ health during periods of decreased circulation.

PROCEDURES USED TO TREAT CARDIOGENIC SHOCK

The most important consideration in cardiogenic shock is to treat the underlying cause. If the cause was an acute MI, then stent placement or emergent CABG should be done. If the shock is a result of papillary muscle rupture, a valve replacement should be considered. If the shock is a result of a ventricular septal defect, repair of the intraventricular septum should be done emergently.

If the patient is having difficulty maintaining adequate oxygenation, the patient should be sedated and intubated. An intra-aortic balloon pump should be placed to decrease cardiac workload and encourage forward movement of blood.

A central line should be placed for multiple medication administration and fluid resuscitation. An arterial line should be considered for more accurate blood pressure management.

MEDICATIONS USED TO MANAGE CARDIOGENIC SHOCK

Vasopressors are given intravenously to help manage hypotension. Typically, these medications are titrated to maintain a mean arterial blood pressure greater than 60 or 65 mm Hg. Dopamine or Dobutamine are often chosen because they also have a positive inotropic effect.

If the patient's blood pressure is able to tolerate it, nitroglycerine is given intravenously to help decrease cardiac workload and increase cardiac output. Analgesics such as intravenous morphine or fentanyl are given for patient comfort and to lower preload.

Diuretics are given to help manage fluid volume and decrease preload; intravenous Lasix is a common medication for this purpose. Natrecor may also be given to reduce preload. Care must be taken in administering these medications as they may also cause hypotension.

CARDIOMYOPATHY

CLASSIFICATIONS OF CARDIOMYOPATHY

There are four major classifications of cardiomyopathy (inflammation of the heart muscle), with each categorized by the etiology of the deterioration. In primary cardiomyopathy, there is no other associated condition and the heart is the only organ affected. Secondary cardiomyopathy is diagnosed when an underlying disease process has affected the heart, such as rheumatic fever, hypertension, valve disease, etc. Ischemic cardiomyopathy results when a coronary artery occlusion deprives the heart of blood, causing the cardiomyopathy. Finally, non-ischemic cardiomyopathy includes the four cardiac muscle conditions list below:

1. Dilated cardiomyopathy, which occurs when damage to the myofibrils (contractile fibers within muscles cells) of the heart cause the left ventricle to become dilated and weak.
2. Hypertrophic cardiomyopathy, which occurs when disease within the heart muscle causes the heart to enlarge (most commonly at the septum), with the septal hypertrophy often decreasing blood flow from the left ventricle into the aorta.
3. Restrictive cardiomyopathy (the rarest of the cardiomyopathies), which results from stiffened ventricular walls.

4. Arrhythmogenic right ventricular cardiomyopathy, which occurs when fat or fibrous tissue replaces heart muscle tissue in the right ventricle (also called arrhythmogenic Right Ventricular Dysplasia (ARVD)).

DILATED CARDIOMYOPATHY

CAUSES

Dilated cardiomyopathy (DCM) is the most common form of cardiomyopathy, as it has a number of potential causes. Many DCM cases are idiopathic (cause unknown). Known causes include vascular abnormalities, such as cardiac ischemia or hypertension. Metabolic causes include diabetes, uremia, thyrotoxicosis, and acromegaly. Other causes include atherosclerosis, heart valve disease, muscular dystrophy, genetics (familial DCM), and childbirth (peripartum DCM), among many others. Viral infections, particularly adenovirus, Varicella zoster, HIV, and Hepatitis C may cause DCM.

DCM may also be seen in patients with alcohol poisoning or cocaine addiction. Those who have been subjected to radiation or heavy metal poisoning, specifically cobalt, are also at risk. Obstetric patients are particularly at risk if they are African American, or have multiparity.

PHYSIOLOGICAL CHANGES

Dilated cardiomyopathy (DCM) often occurs concurrent with extensive coronary artery disease. Poor cardiac perfusion leads to the death of many cardiac muscle cells, which are replaced by scar tissue. The remaining cardiac cells (myocytes) are forced to over-compensate, and thus they become hypertrophied (thickened) and increasingly stretched in coping with overall blood volume. Myocytic contractility increases as the stretching increases, but only to a final compensation threshold. Eventually the muscle cells become stretched beyond compensation, and a dilated (over-stretched) chamber results. The outcome is a weak chamber, unable to properly contract and move blood, causing a decrease in stroke volume and cardiac output. Cardiac size continues to increase as DCM progresses, with the end result being enlargement of the mitral and tricuspid valves and severe valve regurgitation.

SIGNS AND SYMPTOMS

Patients presenting with dilated cardiomyopathy (DCM) typically show signs and symptoms of decreased cardiac output and congestive heart failure. This includes dyspnea and tachycardia while at rest, fatigue, as well as signs of decreased perfusion. Extra heart sounds, such as an S_3 or S_4, may be auscultated. If the disease process has progressed to the point of mitral or tricuspid valve involvement, a holosystolic murmur will be noted. Wheezing or crackles may be heard in the lungs, and pleural effusions may be visualized on a chest X-ray. If the DCM involves the right ventricle, peripheral edema, jugular venous distension, and ascites will be noted.

CLINICAL TESTS TO DIAGNOSE

Dilated cardiomyopathy (DCM) can be diagnosed through a number of tests. An ECG may be done to assess for tachycardia, which is a compensatory mechanism to offset decreased cardiac output. ST segment changes may also be visualized on an ECG.

A chest X-ray can be done to diagnose the associated signs of cardiomegaly. 2D echocardiography can also be used to visualize the increased cardiac size and capture signs and sounds of valvular regurgitation. It can also be used to measure the associated decrease in cardiac ejection fraction. A cardiac catheterization can be done to rule out congestive heart failure.

Lab tests are done to ascertain the source of the cardiomyopathy. These include liver function studies, BUN and creatinine, complete blood count, HIV screening, and thyroid function tests.

HYPERTROPHIC CARDIOMYOPATHY

PATHOPHYSIOLOGY

Hypertrophic cardiomyopathy (HCM) is defined as an idiopathic thickening of the heart muscle, primarily involving the ventricular septum and portions of the left ventricle. Patients with HCM have a genetic disorder that causes them to produce abnormal sarcomeres, or contractile elements. In addition, the normal alignment of muscle cells is absent, resulting in what is called "myocardial disarray." The abnormal sarcomeres are typically the result of a genetic disorder that causes abnormal coding during the production of essential sarcomeric proteins. These abnormal cells become highly concentrated on the ventricular septal wall, decreasing volume capacity and potentially creating an obstruction between the left ventricle and the aorta.

In sum, HCM is characterized by ventricular hypertrophy, an asymmetrical septum, forceful systole and cardiac dysrhythmias, and myocardial disarray.

CAUSES

Hypertrophic cardiomyopathy is primarily caused by a genetic disorder that creates a mutation in the gene responsible for sarcomere production. Approximately 90% of the recorded cases of HCM are caused by this genetic defect.

However, HCM can also be caused by mitochondrial disease, which can affect the 'powerhouse' of the myocytes. Another cause is Anderson-Fabry disease, which is a hereditary deficiency of a lysosomal enzyme. This disease can precipitate HCM by depositing glycosphingolipids in the myocardium, valves, and cardiac conduction system. Obese people have a higher risk of developing HCM. Young athletes are also at risk, and should be closely monitored as they are also at the greatest risk for sudden cardiac death. Patients with Noonan's syndrome, Friedrich's ataxia, or LEOPARD syndrome are also at risk for developing HCM.

SIGNS AND SYMPTOMS

Depending of the extent of the hypertrophy and the age of the patient, symptoms can be minimal or even nonexistent. The abnormal sarcomeres develop gradually over time. It is common for HCM to remain undiagnosed until a patient is aged of fifty or older.

At the time of diagnosis, a patient may present with exertional or atypical chest pain, and dyspnea at rest. The patient may also complain of syncope secondary to cardiac dysrhythmias or decreased cardiac output. Patients with HCM frequently complain of palpitations, and the presence of reoccurring dysrhythmias can be seen on the ECG.

DIAGNOSTIC TOOLS USED TO DIAGNOSE

A detailed family history can be key to diagnosing HCM. Any family history involving myocardial hypertrophy, sudden cardiac death, or reoccurring dysrhythmias should be investigated for HCM.

2D echocardiography is the primary method of diagnosing HCM. Using a 2D echo, structural abnormalities such as ventricular hypertrophy or an asymmetrical intraventricular septum can be visualized. The cardiac ejection fraction can also be measured using a 2D echo.

Pathological Q waves on an ECG may also indicate HCM. A chest X-ray may show cardiomegaly secondary to ventricular hypertrophy. Further, a 48-hour Holter monitor can be worn to monitor and assess the distinctive dysrhythmias caused by HCM.

SURGICAL TREATMENTS

Surgery is indicated for patients with compromised cardiac output secondary to an asymmetrical septum. A septal myectomy can be done to remove the septal muscle portion that is causing the obstruction. Post-surgical mortality is high (3 to 10%), but the procedure can help considerably in relieving symptoms of decreased cardiac output.

An alternate way to treat a septal obstruction is through an alcohol-based septal ablation. This procedure can be done while the patient is under general anesthetic. 100% ethanol is injected into the branch of the left anterior descending artery responsible for supplying the septum with oxygenated blood. This creates an effect similar to a myocardial infarction, causing cell death and consequently thinning the septum.

RESTRICTIVE CARDIOMYOPATHY

PATHOPHYSIOLOGY

Restrictive cardiomyopathy (RCM) occurs when the ventricles become stiff and noncompliant, resulting in decreased end-diastolic cardiac refill volume. The ventricular stiffening is caused by the infiltration of fibroelastic tissue into the cardiac muscle (such as in amyloidosis or sarcoidosis). This leads to heart failure secondary to the decrease in preload and end-diastolic volume.

Atrial enlargement can be seen in most cases of RCM as a result of the increased effort required to push blood from the atria into the ventricles. Some hypertrophy of the ventricles may be noted, but there are generally no changes in the interior dimensions of the ventricle.

SIGNS AND SYMPTOMS

Patients in the early stages of restrictive cardiomyopathy (RCM) typically show no symptoms. However, when the fibroelastic tissue buildup decreases end-diastolic volume, right or left sided heart failure can occur.

Patients with RCM typically present with complaints of exercise intolerance and fatigue. When the right ventricle is affected, peripheral edema, crackles and elevated central venous pressure will be noted. When the left ventricle is affected, extra heart sounds such as an S_3 sound or a murmur will be noted, accompanied by dyspnea while at rest.

It is not uncommon for a patient to be in atrial fibrillation secondary to atrial enlargement. In advanced cases, ventricular dysrhythmias may also be seen.

TESTS USED TO DIAGNOSE

2D echocardiography is the test that is most definitive in diagnosing RCM. It may reveal structural and functional abnormalities in the heart, such as enlarged atria or decreased compliance of the ventricular wall.

Hemodynamic monitoring may also indicate RCM. In RCM, increased right atrial pressures, changes in pulmonary artery pressure as well as in pulmonary artery wedge pressure, and systemic vascular resistance will be seen.

A chest X-ray may indicate cardiomegaly secondary to RCM. An ECG may show atrial fibrillation secondary to RCM.

Because RCM has signs and symptoms similar to constrictive pericarditis, an endomyocardial biopsy can be done during a cardiac catheterization to provide a differential diagnosis.

STRESS-INDUCED CARDIOMYOPATHY

CAUSES AND SYMPTOMS

Stress-induced (Takotsubo) cardiomyopathy results from a sudden surge of catecholamines (such as epinephrine and norepinephrine) in response to a stressful event, such as hypoglycemia, hyperthyroidism, surgery, lightning strike, disaster (earthquake, tornado), death of a family member, or other emotional stress ("broken heart syndrome"). This surge causes a circular ballooning of the left ventricle (similar in shape to the Japanese *tako-tsubo* pot). Stress-induced cardiomyopathy presents differently from those related to coronary artery ischemia. Symptoms are similar to those of an MI and include chest pain typical of angina and dyspnea. In about 20% of cases, the patient develops heart failure. Studies indicate that up to 5% of females diagnosed with MI may, in fact, have stress-induced cardiomyopathy. Stress-induced cardiomyopathy differs from other types of cardiomyopathy in that it usually resolves within 1 to 4 weeks with supportive treatment and rarely results in death or serious morbidity. While stress-induced cardiomyopathy is most common in post-menopausal women (ages 58-75), dilated cardiomyopathy is most common in middle aged males, and hypertrophic cardiomyopathy and restrictive cardiomyopathy in children and young adults.

DIAGNOSTIC PROCEDURES AND TREATMENT OPTIONS

Stress-induced (Takotsubo) cardiomyopathy can be easily misdiagnosed because of lack of familiarity with the disorder and the similarity of symptoms to those of a myocardial infarction. Diagnostic procedures and findings consistent with Takotsubo cardiomyopathy include:

Test	Findings with stress-induced cardiomyopathy
ECG	Elevation of ST segment, marked anterior T-wave inversion, prolonged QT interval, sinus tachycardia.
Cardiac enzymes	Show rapid increase initially but levels fall very quickly.
Echo-cardiogram	LV apical dyskinesia with ballooning of left ventricle.
Cardiac angiography	Coronary artery disease is not significant and does not appear to be related to the cardiomyopathy.
Chest x-ray	Usually normal although may indicate pulmonary edema.

Treatment options generally include oxygen administration to relieve dyspnea and beta-blockers and ACE inhibitors until the left ventricle recovers. Aspirin is often given initially until myocardial infarction is ruled out. If heart failure occurs or other rare complications (ventricular rupture, VT, and mitral regurgitation) then further treatment may be indicated.

MEDICALLY MANAGING CARDIOMYOPATHY

Cardiomyopathy is primarily managed by alleviating cardiac workload. The patient should be placed on adjunctive oxygen when O_2 saturations are less than 90%. Continuous ECG monitoring should be used to monitor for dysrhythmias. If possible, a Swan-Ganz catheter should be inserted to closely monitor hemodynamic function. An intra-aortic balloon pump (IABP) may also be placed to encourage forward blood flow. Diuretics, ACE inhibitors, Beta-blockers, and digoxin may be prescribed as needed to help decrease cardiac workload.

The patient should be encouraged to do small amounts of exercise as their symptoms allow, as exercise can lead to improved oxygen intake and a better quality of life. The patient's fluid and sodium intake should be closely monitored, and limited if necessary.

CONGENITAL HEART DEFECT

A congenital heart defect arises when a heart forms abnormally during fetal development. Congenital heart defects are typically identified and surgically treated when the patient is an infant. However, some birth defects remain unidentified until a patient has reached adulthood. Patients with congenital heart defects may have a malformed septum, such as a complete atrioventricular canal or other less significant ventricular or atrial septal defects. Others may have malformed cardiac valves or arteries, resulting in diagnoses such as aortic valve insufficiency, pulmonary stenosis, or coarctation of the aorta. Other congenital heart defects include Tetralogy of Fallot, Truncus Arteriosus, and Ebstein's anomaly.

> **Review Video: Pediatric Cardiology & Cardiac Defects**
> Visit mometrix.com/academy and enter code: 674392

COARCTATION OF THE AORTA AND TETRALOGY OF FALLOT

Coarctation in the aorta is a narrowing of the aorta between the upper extremities and the lower extremities. This causes increased blood pressure in the upper body. It is typically treated by surgically removing the narrowed potion of the artery.

Tetralogy of Fallot is characterized by four congenital heart defects, with three that occur at the same time. The first of these is a ventricular septal defect (VSD) around the superior aspect of the ventricular septum. Second is an "overriding aorta," so called as it attaches over the VSD defect, allowing both the right and left ventricles to deliver blood into the aorta. Blood from the right ventricle, however, is not oxygenated. The third defect is pulmonary stenosis, where a narrowing of the pulmonary valve and associated structures constrains blood flow to the lungs. The fourth feature is right ventricular hypertrophy, which is actually a secondary condition due to the pulmonary stenosis. Oxygenated blood mixes freely with unoxygenated blood, causing heart failure. Once the condition is discovered, it is typically repaired through a series of surgeries that includes replacement of the pulmonary valve and repair of the ventricular septal defect.

ATRIAL SEPTAL DEFECT VS. COMPLETE ATRIOVENTRICULAR CANAL

An atrial septal defect is a hole in the intra-atrial septum that allows oxygenated blood in the left atrium to mix with unoxygenated blood in the right atrium. Once detected, the patency can then be surgically repaired.

Patients with an atrioventricular canal have an atrial septal defect, a ventricular septal defect, and malformed mitral and tricuspid valves. The additional cardiac workload caused by the shunting of oxygenated blood to the right heart causes heart failure in infants. Surgical treatment involves the repair of the septal defects and replacement of the affected valves.

TRUNCUS ARTERIOSUS AND EBSTEIN'S ANOMALY

Truncus Arteriosus occurs when the embryological "truncus arteriosus" structure fails to divide at its base into the pulmonary artery (leaving the right ventricle) and the aorta (leaving from the left ventricle). Positioned over a ventricular septal defect, it allows both oxygenated and unoxygenated blood to enter. The upper portion of the truncus arteriosus subsequently bifurcates (divides) into the aorta and pulmonary artery, but now it carries mixed blood from both ventricles which leads to heart failure. It is treated by surgically repairing the ventricular septal defect separating the two arteries.

Ebstein's anomaly occurs when the tricuspid valve is malformed, causing one or two of the valve leaflets to be displaced downward into the right ventricle, with a third (often overly large) leaflet potentially adhering to the wall of the ventricle. This causes severe regurgitation (i.e., back flow) between these two chambers. In addition to a malformed tricuspid valve, the patient also typically has an atrial septal defect. The condition is repaired by replacing the tricuspid valve and repairing the atrial septal defect.

CONGENITAL HEART DEFECT IN ADULTS

DIAGNOSIS

If a congenital heart defect is suspected, it can be diagnosed using an echocardiogram. This can detect any structural abnormalities within the heart. Because this is a noninvasive test, it should be considered before any invasive testing.

A cardiac catheterization will also help to detect a congenital heart defect. During the procedure, an angiogram can be taken to visualize the heart directly, and pressures in the cardiac chambers and arteries can be checked using the tip of the catheter.

An ECG can be done to diagnose any cardiac dysrhythmias associated with a congenital heart defect. A chest X-ray may show cardiomegaly, which can occur as a result of a heart defect.

POTENTIAL COMPLICATIONS

Patients with a history of a congenital heart defect are at risk for a number of complications. They are at an increased risk for developing pulmonary hypertension and cardiac dysrhythmias. Further, because patients with a congenital heart defect have abnormal valves, they are also at risk for developing infective endocarditis. The patient is also at increased risk for a stroke as a result of the potential for thrombus formation in and around any defects and their valves.

Though many congenital heart defects are diagnosed and treated when the patient is an infant, some can go undetected until the patient reaches adulthood. A congenital heart defect should be suspected in patients who develop cardiac arrhythmias, cyanosis, shortness of breath, activity intolerance, dizziness, and/or peripheral edema.

TREATMENT

Patients who do not show symptoms related to congenital heart defect may simply be treated with anticoagulation therapy to prevent thrombus formation. Coumadin or Heparin is typically used for this purpose.

Symptomatic adult patients may require surgical treatment of their congenital anomaly. This may involve repair of a septal defect, or a valve replacement.

It may also be necessary to treat the complications of the congenital defect. This may include prescribing antiarrhythmics to prevent cardiac dysrhythmias, or medication therapy for pulmonary hypertension. The patient may also require prophylactic antibiotics prior to any surgeries or invasive treatments to prevent the onset of infective endocarditis.

TEACHING FOR PATIENTS

Patients with a history of a congenital heart defect must be taught that they are at increased risk for life threatening complications as a result of their heart defect. Strict adherence to medication therapy should be stressed. The patient should be encouraged to eat foods that are low in sodium and fat, and to avoid a sedentary lifestyle. The patient should also be encouraged to regularly follow up with their primary care physician. Finally, the patient should also schedule regular dental checkups to prevent endocarditis from developing as a result of an otherwise undetected dental infection.

HYPERTENSION

The normal blood pressure in a healthy adult is composed of a systolic blood pressure less than 120 mm Hg (millimeters of mercury) and a diastolic blood pressure less than 80 mm Hg. When a patient has hypertension, their resting blood pressure measures are greater than these normal levels.

In pre-hypertension, the patient's blood pressure is not yet high enough to have lasting effect, but treatment should be considered to prevent any further increase in blood pressure. A patient with pre-hypertension has a resting systolic blood pressure of 120 to 139 mm Hg and a resting diastolic blood pressure of 80 to 89 mm Hg.

Hypertension is divided into two stages, based upon degrees of risk for additional complications. Stage 1 hypertension is a resting systolic blood pressure in the range of 140 to 159 mm Hg, and a resting diastolic blood pressure of 90 to 99 mm Hg. Stage 2 hypertension is a resting systolic blood pressure greater than 160 mm Hg and a resting diastolic blood pressure greater than 100 mm Hg.

> **Review Video: Hypertension**
> Visit mometrix.com/academy and enter code: 999599

SIGNS AND SYMPTOMS

Patients with hypertension rarely show any signs or symptoms. Some might experience blurred vision, headache, dizziness, or shortness of breath as a result of a sudden elevation of blood pressure. Otherwise, the symptoms are largely silent.

Because hypertension rarely shows symptoms, the first indication is typically organ impairment secondary to hypertension. This can include chest pain as a result of cardiac damage, neurological changes as a result of stroke, or shortness of breath as a result of kidney damage. The patient may also experience vision impairment as a result of damage to the retinas. Often this damage is irreversible, and will require medical management.

PRIMARY, SECONDARY, AND "WHITE COAT" HYPERTENSION

Primary hypertension is an elevated blood pressure with no clear cause as to why it is elevated. This is also referred to as idiopathic hypertension. It is the most common type of hypertension.

Secondary hypertension occurs when problems with other body systems cause an elevation in the blood pressure. The most common cause of secondary hypertension is kidney disease. Secondary hypertension could also be caused by atherosclerotic plaque buildup within the vascular system, sleep apnea, or cancer.

"White coat hypertension" is when a patient's blood pressure is only elevated when taken in a health care setting. It is a feature of anxiety in a clinical setting. Patients with white coat hypertension tend to have a lower blood pressure when it is taken in a non-healthcare setting. Certain patient populations, such as those with diabetes and African-American females are more susceptible to white coat hypertension.

RISK FACTORS

Patients with a family history of hypertension are at an increased risk of developing it themselves. Males are at an increased risk, as are African Americans, pregnant women, people over the age of 35, or people who are obese. Women who are taking oral contraceptives are at an increased risk for developing hypertension. Patients with a previous diagnosis of kidney disease or diabetes should also be carefully monitored for hypertension. Lifestyle choices such as smoking, a sedentary lifestyle, a diet heavy in salt or fatty foods or increased alcohol consumption will increase a person's risk for hypertension.

MALIGNANT HYPERTENSION

Malignant hypertension, or hypertensive crisis, is the sudden rise of blood pressure over a relatively short period of time. Malignant hypertension is characterized by a diastolic blood pressure greater than 140 mm Hg. It can be seen in patients with eclampsia, acute renal failure, or those who abuse cocaine or amphetamines.

Patients with malignant hypertension may experience dizziness, nausea, vision impairment, or renal failure. Blood pressure must be treated quickly to prevent a cerebral vascular accident. Care must be taken to avoid lowering the blood pressure too quickly, as this can lead to cerebral hypoperfusion in patients who have physically acclimated to living with high blood pressure.

TREATMENT

Close blood pressure monitoring is the key to treating malignant hypertension. Placement of an arterial line should be considered; if one is unable to be placed, the patient's peripheral blood pressure should be checked frequently. The patient should be placed on bed rest during the hypertensive crisis. Intravenous vasodilators such as Nipride (sodium nitroprusside) can be given to control blood pressure. Care must be taken, however, as this medication can cause hypokalemia.

Once the hypertensive crisis has passed, blood pressure should be carefully monitored to ensure that it stays within acceptable parameters. Teaching should be done regarding appropriate diet and lifestyle changes to prevent another hypertensive crisis from occurring in the future.

TEACHING FOR A PATIENT

The goal of teaching is to empower the patient to take steps to maintain his blood pressure within a safe range to prevent damage to bodily organs. The patient should be taught to take their medications at appropriate times, and to closely monitor their blood pressure using a home blood pressure monitoring unit.

The patient must also take steps to change their lifestyle. This includes exercising more often, and eating a diet that is low in fat and sodium. If the patient smokes, they should be encouraged to quit, as this leads to worsening of hypertension. The patient should also be taught methods to manage their stress.

HYPERLIPIDEMIA
CAUSES AND IMPACT ON CARDIAC FUNCTION

Hyperlipidemia, particularly increased low-density lipoproteins (LDL), decreased high density lipoproteins (HDL), and increased triglycerides are associated with increased risk of coronary heart disease, especially with other risk factors, such as hypertension, diabetes mellitus, older age, male gender, and history of smoking. The causes of hyperlipidemia may include a number of additional factors, including genetic factors, high fat diet, obesity, and excessive intake of alcohol. Some other disorders, such renal disease and hypothyroidism, are also associated with hyperlipidemia. LDL increases atherosclerosis by accumulating in plagues on the walls of vessels, leading to impaired circulation and risk of clot formation. HDL, on the other hand, transports excess cholesterol to the liver so it can be broken down and excreted. Triglycerides are carried by chylomicron (reflect fat intake after a meal) and very-low density lipoprotein (VLDL) (increased when fasting and reflect carbohydrate intake). After VLDL releases triglycerides for energy, they eventually become LDL with small particles that increase risk of cardiovascular events. Both VLDL and chylomicrons increase inflammation of arterial endothelium.

LAB VALUES THAT INDICATE HYPERLIPIDEMIA

The NIH, NHLBI Report of the National Cholesterol Education Program Expert Panel on Detection, Evaluation, and Treatment of high Blood Cholesterol in Adults classifies total cholesterol, LDL, and HDL to help to determine the need for treatment. Classification includes:

LDL cholesterol	< 100 = Optimal 100 − 129 = Near optimal 130 − 159 = Borderline high 160 − 189 = High ≥ 190 = Very high
Total cholesterol	< 200 = Optimal 200 − 239 = Borderline high ≥ 240 = High
HDL cholesterol	< 40 = Low ≥ 60 = High (optimal)
Triglycerides	< 150 = Normal 150 − 199 = Borderline − high 200 − 499 = High ≥ 500 = Very high

The optimal LDL goal for those with CHD or equivalent risk is < 100 mg/dL; 0-1 risk factors, <160 mg/dL; and more than 2 risk factors, <160 mg/dL. Those with coronary heart disease or equivalent risk factor have a risk of having major coronary events at the rate of >20% per 10 years.

THERAPEUTIC INTERVENTIONS

HMG-CoA REDUCTASE INHIBITORS (STATINS)

Inhibit an enzyme necessary for production of cholesterol, reduce synthesis in the liver, and increase hepatic LDL receptors (which increase uptake and reduce circulating LDL). High intensity statins (such as atorvastatin) reduce LDL by up to 50% while moderate intensity statins (such as fluvastatin) reduce LDL up to 30% with lesser effects on increasing HDL and lowering triglycerides:

- Atorvastatin (Lipitor®) 10-80 mg q day: ≤40% LDL, ≤10% HDL, <<Triglycerides.
- Fluvastatin (Lescol®) 20-40 mg q day: ≤20% LDL, ≤10% HDL, <Triglycerides.
- Lovastatin (Mevacor®) 10-80 mg divided doses: ≤40% LDL, ≤10% HDL, <Triglycerides.
- Pitavastatin (Livalo®) 2-4 mg q day: ≤40% LDL, ≤25% HDL, <<Triglycerides.
- Pravastatin (Pravachol®) 20-80 mg q day: ≤40% LDL, ≤10% HDL, <Triglycerides.
- Rosuvastatin (Crestor®)10-40 mg q day: ≤50% LDL, ≤15% HDL, <<Triglycerides.
- Simvastatin (Zocor®) 5-80 mg q day: ≤40% LDL, ≤10% HDL, <<Triglycerides.

EZETIMIBE

Inhibits absorption of dietary and biliary cholesterol through intestinal wall, reducing LDL by up to 20% or more (if used in combined therapy). Dosage is 10 mg daily.

BILE ACID BINDING RESINS

Bind bile acids in the intestines, decreasing absorption and causing the liver to use hepatic cholesterol to increase production of bile acids to compensate, lowering circulating LDL. Have no effect on triglycerides:

- Cholestyramine (Questran®) 8-24 g divided doses: ≤25% LDL, ≤5% HDL.
- Colesevelam (Welchol®) 3750 mg once daily or in divided doses: ≤20% LDL, ≤10% HDL.
- Colestipol (Colestid®) 10-30 g divided doses: ≤25% LDL, ≤5% HDL.

FIBRIC ACID DERIVATIVES

Reduce plasma triglycerides up to 40%, increase HDL up to 20%, and reduce LDL up to 20%. Used primarily to treat elevated triglycerides:

- Fenofibrate (Tricor®, Antara®, Lipofen®, Fenoglide®, Triglide®) 48-145 mg q day (dosages may vary slightly from one brand to another).
- Gemfibrozil (Lopid®) 600 q day to 600 BID.

DIET

Low fat diet limits saturated and trans fats and encourage fruits, vegetables, lean protein meat, nuts, and whole grains with limited refined carbohydrates and increased fiber. Effects on cholesterol levels vary but reduce LDL by up to 10% for most patients.

ENDOCARDITIS

CAUSES

Endocarditis is an infection of the endothelium of the heart, which includes the heart valves and intraventricular septum. It is the result of bacterial colonization, usually lodging in a previously damaged portion of the endocardium, causing vegetative growth and inflammation. Infective endocarditis is typically caused by Streptococcus or Staphylococcus bacterium.

Intravenous drug abuse is one of the primary causes of infective endocarditis; patients in this particular population are most at risk for fungal endocarditis. Infective endocarditis is also seen in cases of rheumatic valvular disease and congenital heart disease. It can also occur after valve replacement surgery.

SIGNS AND SYMPTOMS

Patients with infective endocarditis typically present with a low-grade fever and the presence of a murmur from the affected valve. The patient may also present with lesions of the hands or fingers, referred to as Janeway lesions or Osler nodes, respectively. Further, patients may present with signs and symptoms of heart failure secondary to valvular insufficiency or regurgitation. This may include shortness of breath, jugular venous distension, crackles in the lungs, and/or peripheral edema.

A significant portion of the patients who present with signs of infective endocarditis also present with neurological sequelae, such as stroke or brain abscess, as a result of thrombi that form on the vegetative growth on the valves and later become dislodged.

SUBACUTE BACTERIAL ENDOCARDITIS

Subacute bacterial endocarditis (SBE) is a rare condition seen after an invasive procedure (usually in the mouth or throat, such as tooth extraction or tonsillectomy) is performed on a patient who has valvular heart disease (i.e., an abnormal valve or a damaged valve). SBE occurs when the patient acquires a bacterial infection in the blood. The bacteria adhere to the fibrin and platelets present on the previously damaged valve. If left untreated, it can prove fatal within six months after the onset of symptoms.

The patient may initially present with mild symptoms, including a low-grade fever and chest pain. SBE can rapidly progress to heart failure as the bacteria adhered to the valve forms vegetation. Intensive antibiotic therapy should be provided as quickly as possible to prevent deterioration. If the patient already has a history of heart failure secondary to valvular heart disease, an emergent valve replacement should be considered.

DIAGNOSIS AND TREATMENT

A number of tests can be helpful in diagnosing infective endocarditis. A transthoracic echocardiogram (TTE) can be done to assess valve function and display any vegetation that may be present. In cases of acute endocarditis, the patient will have an elevated erythrocyte sedimentation rate and C-reactive protein level.

The key to diagnosing infective endocarditis is identifying the microbe responsible for the infection so that the appropriate course of treatment can be initiated. Blood cultures are the most definite way of determining the microbe responsible for endocarditis.

A CT scan of the head should be done to rule out cerebral vascular accident in any patients showing neurological changes.

MYOCARDITIS

Myocarditis refers to a collection of inflammatory processes that affect the cardiac muscle. It is characterized by inflammation of the myocytes, and, with subsequent myocytic necrosis, and may lead to congestive heart failure or dilated cardiomyopathy. Myocarditis can affect any patient population, but is most prevalent among healthy adult males.

In myocarditis, an initial insult affects the cardiac tissue, such as exposure to a disease process or a toxic substance. This insult causes damage to the cardiac muscle, initiating an immune response. In the case of myocarditis, the immune response is overactive, causing destruction of the myocytes as well as the antigen that triggered the immune response.

CAUSES

Myocarditis can be caused by a number of pathogens and toxic substances, and these are typically categorized as infectious and noninfectious causes.

Infectious causes can be viral, bacterial, or fungal. Potential viral pathogens include Rubella, Polio, Influenza, Adenovirus, HIV, and Hepatitis B. Common bacterial pathogens include Legionella, Diphtheria, Salmonella, or Pseudomonas. Fungal causes include Candidiasis, Aspergillosis, and Blastomycosis.

Certain systemic diseases and autoimmune processes can also cause myocarditis. These can include Lupus Erythematosus, Sarcoidosis, Crohn's disease, and Thyrotoxicosis. Myocarditis can also be seen during the rejection process following a heart transplant.

Drug induced causes of myocarditis include cocaine and alcohol abuse, arsenic, and catecholamines.

SIGNS AND SYMPTOMS

Myocarditis can be difficult to diagnose because of the many potential causes, and because symptoms may vary widely from patient to patient. Some patients may only experience flu-like symptoms, while others show signs and symptoms of congestive heart failure. However, there are some symptoms that are consistent in all cases of myocarditis.

Patients with myocarditis typically complain of chest pain, and exhibit dyspnea. They also typically have a low-grade fever, and symptoms of syncope, fatigue, malaise, and palpitations. Soft heart sounds, extra heart sounds such as S3, mitral or tricuspid valve murmurs, or a friction rub may be auscultated. The patient may be hypotensive or exhibit tachycardia. Signs of fluid overload such as crackles in the lungs, jugular venous distension, or peripheral edema may also be noted.

DIAGNOSIS

Magnetic resonance imaging (MRI) is helpful in diagnosing myocarditis because is reveals areas of inflammation. These appear as "patchy" areas on an MRI. If myocarditis was previously suspected, a biopsy can be done during the MRI to obtain tissue samples for definitive testing.

A 2D echo can also be done to show cardiac structural or functional abnormalities, such as decreased ventricular wall motion or decreased ejection fraction. Using a 2D echo, pericardial effusions may also be visualized.

An ECG can be done to help provide a differential diagnosis from acute MI. During myocarditis, ST segment elevations will be noted, but there will be no reciprocal lead changes.

TREATMENT

The goal of treatment is to identify the underlying cause of the myocarditis and provide appropriate care. If the infection is bacterial or fungal, antibiotics or antifungals may be required. If the cause is drug induced, identification and removal of the offending substance is necessary.

Accompanying signs and symptoms should also be treated accordingly. Fluid overload and congestive heart failure treatment includes the administration of diuretics to manage fluid status, and the use of ACE inhibitors, beta-blockers, and calcium channel blockers to manage cardiac afterload, as well as cardiac glycosides to improve contractility.

Adjunctive oxygen may be necessary to decrease cardiac workload. If the patient becomes febrile, steps must be taken to lower their temperature.

PERICARDITIS

CAUSES

Pericarditis is an inflammatory response that takes place in the pericardium. It is typically caused by an infectious process, or as a complication of an acute myocardial infarction. Viral infections are the most common cause of infectious pericarditis. The various infectious pathogens can include Coxsackie virus, pseudomonas, or aspergillosis.

Pericarditis can also be seen after an acute MI. This is referred to as Dressler's syndrome. It occurs most commonly after an anterior wall MI, as it involves the largest area of the heart. The presence of extravascular blood or necrotic tissue triggers the inflammatory response.

Other causes of pericarditis include uremia, trauma, or systemic conditions such as sarcoidosis or lupus erythematosus.

SIGNS AND SYMPTOMS

The most common symptom of pericarditis is chest pain. This pain typically has a sudden onset, and increases in intensity whenever lying flat or taking deep breaths. The patient may experience shortness of breath as a result of inspiratory-restrictive pain while taking deep breaths. The patient may also be diaphoretic as a result of pain intensity. The patient may experience other vague symptoms, such as a low-grade fever (as a result of the triggered immune response), increased anxiety, and restlessness.

The primary clinical sign noted in pericarditis is the presence of a "friction rub" sound on auscultation. The friction rub will remain audible by auscultation even while the patient is holding their breath.

DIAGNOSIS AND TREATMENT

In pericarditis, the patient will show diffuse "saddle-shaped" ST segment elevations, and a depressed PR interval on ECG. A chest X-ray may show an enlarged heart secondary to the inflammation.

Pericarditis is diagnosed by the detection of an elevated white blood cell count in a complete blood count after an acute myocardial infarction. If pericarditis is suspected, an echocardiogram should also be done to assess for cardiac effusions.

Pericarditis is treated with NSAIDs, such as aspirin, to reduce the inflammatory process. If this approach is unsuccessful, the patient may be started on steroids and colchicine in an attempt to reduce the inflammation. The patient may also be given antibiotics if the cause is bacterial or antifungal medications if it is fungal. If the presence of severe cardiac effusion is decreasing preload, pericardiocentesis will be done to decrease the constriction on the heart.

TREATMENT OF ANY ACUTE INFLAMMATORY DISEASE

Direct care of the patient with a diagnosis of any acute inflammatory disease involves the relief of patient symptoms. Bed rest should be encouraged to reduce the amount of stress placed upon the heart. Fever and pain should be treated appropriately. Care should be taken to ensure that antibiotics are given at appropriate intervals, and that adequate serum medication levels are maintained. The patient's fluid balance should be closely monitored, and any electrolyte imbalances should be reported and treated. The patient's vital signs should be closely monitored, and any changes reported immediately, as a patient with myocarditis can deteriorate quickly.

PAPILLARY MUSCLE RUPTURE

Papillary muscle rupture occurs infrequently after AMI (acute myocardial infarction) – occurring in 40% of patients after a posterior septal MI and in 20% of anterior septal MI patients. Symptoms of a papillary muscle rupture include a holosystolic murmur and thrill that radiates to the axilla. This results from severe mitral or tricuspid valve regurgitation. If the tricuspid valve is involved, the patient will experience right-side heart failure. Acute cardiogenic shock and pulmonary edema occur in the case of mitral valve involvement.

Prompt detection of papillary muscle rupture is crucial. Interventions are aimed at increasing adequate perfusion and reducing afterload through the use of intra-aortic balloon pumping, positive inotropes, and vasodilators. The patient should be prepared for an emergent valve replacement surgery.

PERICARDIAL EFFUSION

Pericardial effusion is a collection of fluid, blood, or pus in the pericardium, resulting from pericardial inflammation associated with pericarditis or myocarditis (often viral), malignancies (such as lung and breast cancer and leukemia), heart failure, HIV, chronic renal failure, and post cardiac surgery (especially if chest tube are removed early). Pericardial effusions may be acute with abrupt onset of symptoms (dyspnea, tachycardia, hypotension, anxiety) leading to cardiac tamponade and pulseless electrical activity unless pericardiocentesis is carried out immediately. However, chronic pericardial effusions may be asymptomatic until about 2 L of fluid (normal volume 15 to 50 mL) have accumulated because the slow effusion allows the pericardium to stretch. Patients may demonstrate only dull chest pain, cough, hiccoughs, nausea, and vomiting initially with symptoms slowly increasing. If asymptomatic, the effusion may be treated with NSAIDs and corticosteroids and treatment of underlying cause. If symptoms are severe, then pericardiocentesis may be necessary. With pericardial effusion, the ECG may show reduced voltage with small effusion but electrical alternans (altered QRS complex with sinus tachycardia) with large.

PULMONARY EDEMA

Pulmonary edema is a buildup of fluid in the lungs, causing inadequate oxygen and carbon dioxide exchange. The edema is typically caused by cardiac dysfunction, with congestive heart failure being the primary cause. However, pulmonary edema can be a result of myocardial infarction, cardiomyopathy, pericardial effusions, or a hypertensive crisis, as well.

There are also a variety of non-cardiac causes of pulmonary edema. Patients with a history of recent pneumonia or other lung infections are at greater risk. ARDS (adult respiratory distress syndrome), pulmonary contusion or aspiration can also cause pulmonary edema. Inhalation of toxic substances, such as ammonia, chlorine, or smoke inhalation may cause irritation to the alveoli, which may also cause pulmonary edema.

SIGNS AND SYMPTOMS

Pulmonary edema can develop gradually, or quite suddenly. If the progression is gradual, patients begin showing symptoms of mild fluid overload during the course of a few days or weeks. These symptoms include shortness of breath, peripheral edema, nocturia (getting up frequently at night to pass urine) and weight gain. Some patients may also complain of paroxysmal nocturnal dyspnea (a sudden shortness of breath that develops while sleeping).

Symptoms of severe pulmonary edema include to those listed above, as well as anxiety or restlessness secondary to hypoxia, diaphoresis, wheezing, decreased level of consciousness, and pallor. Pink, frothy sputum is a classic sign of pulmonary edema.

DIAGNOSIS

A complete medical history can provide clues to aid in the diagnosis of pulmonary edema. It should be suspected in any patient with a history significant of myocardial infarction, valvular heart disease, or congestive heart failure (CHF).

An arterial blood gas (ABG) may be done to assess the patient's oxygenation. A decreased PO_2 on an ABG indicates a decrease in oxygen perfusion. Blood tests for B-type natriuretic peptide (BNP) may also be used to diagnose CHF. A complete blood count will assess red blood cell count, white blood cell count, hemoglobin, and hematocrit. Electrolytes may be drawn to check levels of sodium and potassium.

The diagnosis of pulmonary edema can be verified with a chest X-ray, where areas of fluid buildup would appear cloudy within the lungs. A 2D echocardiograph may also be done to assess the cause of the pulmonary edema, such as valvular regurgitation, low ejection fraction, or pericardial effusions.

TREATMENT

The primary focus of treating pulmonary edema is to maintain adequate oxygenation. The patient will be placed on adjunctive oxygen or on continuous positive airway pressure (CPAP) in cases of decreased PO_2 combined with increased in CO_2. CPAP forces air into the lungs at a prescribed pressure, reducing pulmonary workload. In cases of severe hypoxia, sedation and mechanical ventilation may be required.

The focus of medical management includes decreasing cardiac workload and achieving an appropriate fluid balance. Diuretics are prescribed for cardiac preload reduction by removing excess fluid from the interstitial tissues and circulatory system. Cardiac workload is also reduced by afterload reduction is using nitrates or ACE inhibitors. Morphine may be given to reduce shortness of breath.

SUDDEN CARDIAC DEATH

Sudden cardiac death (SCD) is due to the abrupt and total loss of cardiac function. Chest pain and other indicators of cardiac dysfunction typically occur within an hour preceding SCD. Loss of consciousness and subsequent death is usually caused by a sudden loss of circulation due to ventricular tachycardia or ventricular fibrillation.

Because there are often few symptoms prior to the onset of SCD, the patient is typically in the community when it occurs. Brain death occurs four to six minutes after the loss of circulation. Without the prompt administration of ACLS protocols, corporeal death usually occurs soon after that.

RISK FACTORS

The primary risk factor for sudden cardiac death (SCD) is coronary artery disease. Studies have shown that at least two major coronary arteries were occluded in 90% of those who died from SCD. Further, 75% of the patients who had SCD also had a previous history of myocardial infarction. In many other cases, those affected by SCD had previously been diagnosed with congestive heart failure or valvular disorders. Other risk factors include cardiomyopathy, Wolff-Parkinson-White (WPW) syndrome, or long QT syndrome.

Statistically, African Americans are at the highest risk for SCD. Men are at greater risk than women. The age group at greatest risk is inclusive of those between 45-75 years of age.

TREATMENT FOR SYMPTOMS

Prompt defibrillation and administration of ACLS protocols is essential for subsequent survival. Because brain death occurs within four to six minutes after loss of circulation, and physical death occurs 10 minutes after loss of circulation, CPR must be initiated immediately. Defibrillation should take place as soon as a defibrillating unit can be made available.

Once the patient arrives at a hospital setting, prompt treatment of the underlying cause should be initiated to prevent further dysrhythmias from occurring. This can include cardiac catheterization, intra-aortic balloon pump (IABP) placement, or the placement of an automatic implantable cardioverter-defibrillator (AICD) device and pacemaker.

Valvular Heart Disease
Causes

It is much more common for valvular heart disease to be acquired over time, though the acquisition time can differ depending upon the cause and which valve is involved. Congenital heart defects account for only a small percentage of valvular heart disease cases.

Rheumatic heart disease and endocarditis can both cause valvular heart disease in all four of the heart's valves. Drugs used to enhance dieting are also responsible for some valvular disease occurrences.

Pulmonary valve disease may be caused by pulmonary hypertension, or by idiopathic dilation of the pulmonary artery.

Aortic valve disease may be caused by aortic dissection, calcified buildup on the valve, or arteriosclerosis.

Myocardial infarction is the chief cause of mitral valve disease. It can also be caused by cardiomyopathy, lupus erythematosus, and mitral valve prolapse.

Tricuspid valve disease may be caused by pulmonary hypertension, mitral valve prolapse, and right heart failure.

Diagnosis

A murmur auscultated over the affected valve is often then first indication of valvular heart disease. There are a number of tests available to diagnose the valvular disorder. A transthoracic echocardiogram (TTE) is typically the first test done, as it is noninvasive. However, visualization can be limited based on body mass and type.

A transesophageal echocardiogram is often the next choice if a TTE is inconclusive. Care must be taken because the test is invasive. Close monitoring of the patient's vital signs is important, as conscious sedation is required to perform the TTE.

Valvular heart disease can also be visualized during a cardiac catheterization. This test carries the most risks of the three because there is a strong risk of complication from bleeding or adverse reactions to the contrast media. It is, however, the most accurate of the three tests.

Mitral Valve
Regurgitation

Mitral valve regurgitation occurs when blood is pushed back into the left atrium from the left ventricle through the closed mitral valve. This is typically caused by the failure of one of the parts of the mitral valve: the chorda tendineae, the mitral annulus, the papillary muscles, or the mitral leaflets.

In chronic mitral regurgitation, atrial hypertrophy can occur as a result of increased pressure during ventricular diastole. Stroke volume decreases as a result of ventricular hypertrophy. Despite compensatory mechanisms, left ventricular failure will occur, eventually followed by right ventricular failure if the condition is left untreated.

In cases of acute mitral regurgitation, there is no time for the initiation of compensatory mechanisms. The onset of left heart failure takes place shortly after the onset of mitral regurgitation.

STENOSIS

Mitral valve stenosis decreases the size of the mitral valve, resulting in an increased amount of pressure required to push blood from the left atrium to the left ventricle during diastole. Pressure in the left atrium increases to prevent backflow of blood into the pulmonary system and right ventricle. This results in hypertrophy of the left atrium.

As mitral valve stenosis worsens, stroke volume of the left ventricle decreases. Contractility and heart rate increase in order to compensate for the lack of forward blood flow. This results in left ventricular hypertrophy. Pulmonary hypertension is also likely to occur.

TREATMENT

Treatment for mitral regurgitation and mitral stenosis is dependent upon the type and severity of symptoms exhibited. Efforts will be taken to provide relief for symptoms of heart failure and decreased cardiac output. If symptoms are unable to be controlled through medical management, valve replacement should be considered.

Atrial fibrillation typically occurs as a result of atrial remodeling to compensate for lack of forward blood flow. If the patient is found to be in A-fibrillation, anticoagulation therapy is an important consideration to prevent thromboembolic disorders. Rate control and cardiac workload are also to be considered; beta-blockers, digoxin or calcium channel blockers may be prescribed for this purpose.

MITRAL VALVE PROLAPSE AND MITRAL VALVE PROLAPSE SYNDROME

Mitral valve prolapse is a weakening in the leaflets of the mitral valve, causing them to bulge upward into the left atrium during ventricular contraction. A systolic click can be auscultated that results as the chordae tendineae are tightly stretched during diastole. Mitral valve prolapse may lead to mitral valve regurgitation if the weakening in the leaflets becomes too pronounced.

Most patients with mitral valve prolapse do not experience any symptoms. However, in some cases, mitral valve prolapse syndrome may occur. Mitral valve prolapse syndrome is when the patient experiences chest pain without the presence of ischemia. The chest pain is typically accompanied with shortness of breath and vertigo. The etiology of mitral valve prolapse syndrome is unknown. It is typically treated with beta-blockers to relieve the chest pain.

AORTIC STENOSIS

In aortic valve stenosis, there is a narrowing of the opening between the left ventricle and the aorta. This requires more ventricular effort to maintain adequate stroke volume, resulting in increased pressure in the left ventricle. Ventricular hypertrophy develops as a result of increased cardiac workload, reducing the volume capacity. This further decreases ventricular stroke volume.

Aortic valve replacement is the treatment of choice for aortic stenosis. While awaiting surgery, nitrates may be used to treat chest pain, and vasodilators may be used to decrease afterload. Adjunctive oxygen may be required to decrease cardiac workload.

AORTIC INSUFFICIENCY

Aortic insufficiency is when there is a weakness in the aortic valve that allows small amounts of blood to flow back into the left ventricle through the closed valve. This creates ventricular remodeling similar to that in aortic stenosis, such as ventricular hypertrophy and a decrease in blood volume capacity. If left untreated, the patient will show symptoms of congestive heart failure or diastolic and systolic heart failure.

Blood pressure control is important for patients who are symptomatic with aortic insufficiency. ACE inhibitors and hydralazine are the medications of choice for treating elevated blood pressure. When clinically stable, it is recommended that an aortic valve replacement be performed.

TRICUSPID VALVE STENOSIS AND REGURGITATION

Tricuspid valve stenosis is the narrowing of the opening between the right atrium and the right ventricle, requiring increased atrial effort to push blood to the ventricle. Tricuspid regurgitation is the backflow of blood from the right ventricle to the right atrium. Both tricuspid stenosis and tricuspid regurgitation can lead to increased pressures in the right atrium and right-sided hypertrophy.

Tricuspid stenosis and tricuspid regurgitation typically occur alongside mitral valve stenosis or regurgitation, usually secondary to rheumatic fever. In most cases, treatment of the mitral valve regurgitation or stenosis is enough to provide relief of symptoms secondary to tricuspid valve difficulties.

PULMONARY STENOSIS AND INSUFFICIENCY

Pulmonary stenosis occurs when there is a narrowing of the pulmonary valve, requiring more effort to move blood from the right ventricle into the pulmonary artery. In pulmonary insufficiency, there is a weakening in the pulmonary valve leaflets, causing blood to flow from the pulmonary artery to the right ventricle.

Pulmonary insufficiency and stenosis take place much less frequently than mitral or aortic valve disease. Even when the pulmonary insufficiency or stenosis is severe, the patient may not show any symptoms. In some severe cases, however, the patient may show signs of right heart failure. Diuretics and digoxin may be prescribed to treat the right-sided heart failure.

VENTRICULAR ANEURYSM

CAUSES

A ventricular aneurysm is an outward ballooning of the ventricular wall. The etiology commonly involves a myocardial infarction secondary to a coronary artery occlusion, resulting in necrosed cardiac tissue in the affected area of the heart. Over time, the necrosed tissue heals and is replaced by scar tissue, leaving a weakened area in the ventricular wall. During diastole, increased ventricular pressure causes the weakened tissue to balloon outward, creating the aneurysm.

The patient may not exhibit symptoms if the aneurysm is small. If the patient does experience symptoms, they usually begin to appear after ventricular remodeling has taken place. This may be three days to several months after the myocardial infarction. Patients with ventricular aneurysm typically present with an S3 gallop, signs and symptoms of heart failure, and ST segment elevations on an ECG.

DIAGNOSIS

Ventricular aneurysm is primarily diagnosed by visualization through left ventriculography during a cardiac catheterization. However, there are a number of noninvasive tests that may indicate the presence of a ventricular aneurysm. An ECG will show ST segment elevations that are present in the absence of chest pain. A 2d echocardiogram or radionuclide ventriculography may show the weakening of the ventricular wall or hemostasis within the aneurysm. It will also show any thrombi that are present within the aneurysm. The bulge of the aneurysm may also be visualized by chest X-ray or an MRI.

COMPLICATIONS

Because the scar tissue lacks the contractility of healthy heart tissue, complications of ventricular aneurysm occur as a result of decreased pumping ability. These include cardiac ischemia and congestive heart failure. The patient may also experience intractable ventricular dysrhythmias, particularly V-tach.

Patients with a ventricular aneurysm are also at risk for thromboembolic disorders, such as acute myocardial infarction, stroke, pulmonary embolus, or peripheral ischemia. Hemostasis can occur within the aneurysm, resulting in the formation of thrombi. Therefore, it is important to place patients with a ventricular aneurysm on anticoagulation therapy as a preventative measure.

VENTRICULAR ANEURYSMECTOMY

A ventricular aneurysmectomy is indicated for patients who are symptomatic with a ventricular aneurysm, particularly if they are showing symptoms of decreased perfusion or intractable V-tach. An aneurysmectomy is done during cardiopulmonary bypass. When the patient is placed on bypass, healthy cardiac tissue remains firm, while the aneurysm collapses inward. An incision is made over the aneurysm, and any thrombi are removed from the ventricle. The edges of the aneurysm are then sutured closed.

After an aneurysmectomy, the patient should be monitored for signs and symptoms of bleeding, respiratory complications and kidney failure. It is important to monitor the patient via continuous ECG, as well as obtaining a complete blood count and chest X-ray.

Surgery is not indicated for patients who do not show any signs or symptoms of decreased cardiac output. However, the patient may require anticoagulation to prevent thrombus formation within the aneurysm.

VENTRICULAR SEPTAL RUPTURE

Ventricular septal rupture (VSR) occurs when a myocardial infarction weakens the septum between the right and left ventricles, resulting in tearing. In consequence, oxygenated blood in the left ventricle is shunted into the right ventricle. Cardiac workload is increased as the right ventricle pumps oxygenated blood to the lungs, leaving the left ventricle with less oxygenated blood to pump into the body.

A patient with VSR typically presents with a new holosystolic murmur that radiates to from the cardiac apex to the axilla, as well as hypotension, congestive heart failure, and shortness of breath. A chest X-ray may show cardiomegaly, and an echocardiogram will show shunting of the blood from the left to right ventricles.

Interventions are aimed at restoring adequate perfusion and reducing afterload through the use of intra-aortic balloon pumping, positive inotropes, and vasodilators. The patient should be prepared for emergent surgery to repair the tear.

Vascular Issues

ACUTE ARTERIAL OCCLUSION

Acute arterial occlusion occurs when there is a sudden decrease or stoppage of arterial blood flow. Blood flow is typically halted to an extremity, but it might also be slowed to the kidneys or other body organs, as well. Blood flow must be returned to the muscle within a short period of time, or the patient will experience rhabdomyolysis. Failure to return circulation or an organ can result in ischemic damage and even organ failure. Acute arterial occlusion is typically caused by an atherosclerotic rupture that obstructs blood flow. Other causes may include a thrombus formation, aortic dissection, or compartment syndrome.

Patients who have hyperlipidemia or hypercholesterolemia are at increased risk for acute arterial occlusion. Patients with diabetes, atrial fibrillation, valve disorders, or those with clotting disorders are also at greater risk.

SIGNS AND SYMPTOMS IN AN EXTREMITY

Acute arterial occlusion is characterized by sharp pain in an extremity as a result of the sudden decrease in oxygenated blood to the muscle. As muscle cells become damaged as a result of lack of oxygenation, the patient may experience numbness or a tingling sensation in the affected limb. In severe cases, the patient may even experience loss of movement. Pulses in the affected limb may be thready, or absent by palpation. The skin distal to the occlusion may become pale, mottled or cyanotic, and will be cool to the touch.

DIAGNOSIS AND TREATMENT

When a patient presents with signs and symptoms of decreased blood flow to an extremity, an arteriogram is done to assess circulation within the extremity. Contrast dye is injected intravenously, which is followed by a series of X-rays in an attempt to visualize any occlusions.

The primary goal of treatment is to restore circulation to the affected extremity as quickly as possible. This can be done through the administration of a thrombolytic such as tPA or Streptokinase. Catheterization and stent placement may be performed to reopen the occluded artery. If the patient is healthy enough, arterial bypass can be performed to surgically remove the occluded area of the artery and replace it with a patent artery. A fasciotomy (tissue incision) may be considered if the affected limb has become profoundly swollen from the loss of circulation for an extended period of time. This will reduce tissue tension and pressure in the affected limb, thereby aiding in circulatory restoration.

CAROTID ARTERY STENOSIS

Carotid artery stenosis refers to the gradual narrowing of the carotid arteries. This is often the result of the buildup of atherosclerotic plaque along the inner lumen of the artery. As the carotid artery narrows, blood flow to the brain is gradually slowed.

Occasionally, the atherosclerotic plaque ruptures, sending small pieces into the bloodstream. This places the patient at risk for ischemic stroke or repeated transient ischemic attacks (TIAs), as the plaque is unable to pass the blood- brain barrier and thus lodges itself within the cerebral capillaries.

Coronary artery disease is the greatest risk factor for coronary artery stenosis. Other risk factors include diabetes, atrial fibrillation, valvular disorder, and cardiomyopathy.

SIGNS AND SYMPTOMS

A patient with carotid artery stenosis typically does not show any symptoms until a stroke or transient ischemic attack (TIA) occurs. Patients who are having a stroke or TIA may experience sudden loss of consciousness, difficulty speaking, or an altered mental status. Physical signs may include generalized weakness, and/or loss of sensation or paralysis on one side of the body. These are typically accompanied by a headache.

In the case of a TIA, the symptoms will remain for a short period of time, typically a few minutes or hours before gradually resolving. TIAs have the same signs and symptoms as a stroke, and often are only diagnosed after the symptoms resolve.

DIAGNOSIS

One indicator of carotid artery stenosis is the presence of a bruit that can be auscultated over the carotid artery. A bruit is a whooshing noise that can be heard as blood passes through a narrowed area in the artery.

A carotid Doppler can be done noninvasively to assess carotid circulation. A Doppler used sound waves to assess the patency of the artery.

An MR-A (magnetic resonance angiography) of the brain is also a noninvasive test that uses contrast dye and magnetic waves to generate detailed images of the cerebral vasculature.

The most common test used to diagnose carotid artery stenosis is the cerebral angiogram. It is an invasive procedure that involves injecting contrast dye intravenously while the doctor monitors live motion X-rays in order to locate any occlusions. The primary risks associated with cerebral angiogram are stroke and bleeding.

VARIOUS TREATMENTS

Medical management of carotid artery stenosis includes the administration of platelet inhibitors such as Aspirin, Plavix, or Coumadin. Care should be taken to make sure that the patient takes an appropriate amount of medication to ensure adequate levels in the bloodstream. If the patient is planning to have any sort of surgery, they should inform their surgeon that they are taking a platelet inhibitor.

A carotid endarterectomy is the most common procedure used to remove atherosclerotic plaque from the interior of an artery. An incision is made over the affected area, and the plaque is excised. The artery is then sewn shut. The patient should be closely monitored for signs and symptoms of bleeding or hematoma following the procedure.

TEACHING FOR A PATIENT

Treatment for carotid artery stenosis includes medication therapy and lifestyle changes. For proper medication management, it is important to take the proper dosages of medication to maintain appropriate blood levels. The patient may also be prescribed lipid-lowering agents to control atherosclerotic plaque buildup. Therefore, teaching includes the necessity for these medicines and their appropriate use.

Lifestyle changes include increasing the amount of exercise, developing healthy eating habits, limiting alcohol consumption, and smoking cessation. Blood pressure should be carefully controlled in patients with a history of hypertension. If the patient has been previously diagnosed with diabetes, it should be carefully managed. Cholesterol levels should be checked regularly. The presence of a bruit should be closely monitored.

VENOUS THROMBOSIS

Venous thrombosis is a blood clot that forms in a vein. The blood clot typically forms through a combination of three factors: decreased activity, damage to a venous valve or vessel wall, and a hypercoagulable state. Venous thrombosis is significant because patients with the condition are at increased risk for developing a pulmonary embolus. Thrombi form primarily in the lower extremities as a result of venous stasis. When a thrombus occurs in an upper extremity, it is typically the result of a blood clot that has formed on a central line. Patients most at risk for developing venous thrombosis are those who have had cancer, stroke, heart failure, and kidney disease.

SIGNS AND SYMPTOMS

The size of the blood clot and extent of the occlusion have a direct relationship to the severity of any signs or symptoms that may occur. If the thrombus is located in a superficial vein with sufficient collateral blood flow, the patient may not display any symptoms.

The classic symptoms of venous thrombosis are pain, swelling and redness in the affected extremity. There may be tenderness along the venous tract. If venous thrombosis is suspected, the Homan's sign can be performed. The patient should be asked to dorsiflex the foot. The presence of pain in the calf indicates the presence of a blood clot. Homan's sign may be inconclusive, however, as it is only present in 50% of the population.

DIAGNOSIS

A positive D-dimer blood test may be indicative of venous thrombosis. An elevated D-Dimer means there is a clot present in the body that is in the process of being broken down. A normal D-dimer level indicates that there are no blood clots actively being broken down in the body.

The presence of a venous thrombosis can be directly confirmed through a Doppler ultrasound or through an MRI of the affected extremity. Both tests are noninvasive. The Doppler can even be done at the bedside, as a portable test. The MRI, however, requires the patient to be moved to the MRI machine, as well as the injection of contrast dye. It is best for locating pelvic thrombi.

TREATMENTS

Because of the elevated risk for pulmonary embolus, the major treatment focus is on the prevention of any venous thrombi before they manifest. The use of sequential compression stockings to deter venous stasis is one way to prevent venous thrombi from forming. The patient may also be encouraged to do leg exercises while in bed. Low molecular weight Heparin or Coumadin may also be administered prophylactically.

Once a venous thrombus has been diagnosed, the patient is typically started on intravenous anticoagulation. If anticoagulation is contraindicated for the patient, or if they have reoccurring venous thrombi, the placement of an inferior vena cava (IVC) filter may be considered to prevent a pulmonary embolus. Pharmacological thrombolysis may also be considered for a large clot.

AORTIC ANEURYSMS

THORACIC AND ABDOMINAL ANEURYSMS

Thoracic aortic aneurysms occur in the chest in the ascending, arch, or descending segments and are often asymptomatic but may cause substernal pain, back pain, dyspnea and/or stridor (from pressure on trachea), cough, distention of neck veins, and edema of neck and arms. Rupture usually does not allow time for emergent repair, so identifying and correcting before rupture is essential. Surgery (a high-risk procedure) is indicated for aneurysms ≥6 cm.

About 90% of **abdominal aortic aneurysms** occur in the lower part of the aorta below the renal arteries, but aneurysms are not usually palpable until they reach 5 cm/diameter, so they may be found incidentally when an abdominal pulsatile mass is noted. Patients may have had mild constant or intermittent pain, but rupture results in severe abdominal pain, hypotension, and a palpable mass. About 50% of patients die with rupture. Elective repair is usually advised for aneurysms >5.5 cm or those that are rapidly expanding.

CAUSES

An aortic aneurysm develops when a portion of the aorta dilates to greater than one and a half times the normal diameter, stretching and weakening the artery wall. Dissection occurs when the wall of the aorta is torn and blood flows between the layers of the wall, dilating and weakening it until it risks rupture (which has a high mortality rate). Dissection most commonly occurs in the thoracic aorta (proximal ascending aorta about 5 cm distal to the aortic valve or descending aorta just distal to the left subclavian artery) although it can occur throughout the aorta. Causes of aortic aneurysm may include atherosclerosis, hypertension, trauma (such as blunt thoracic trauma), infection, cocaine use, syphilis (rare), or genetic defect affecting the collagen or elastin elements of the vasculature, such as Marfan syndrome, Ehlers-Danlos disease, and other connective tissue disorders.

RISK FACTORS

Males have five times higher incidence than females. Other risk factors include age (>60), smoking (especially of long duration, increases risk 8 times), statin use, hypertension, hyperlipidemia, PAD, and family history

DIAGNOSTIC TESTS AND INTERVENTIONS

Diagnosis of **aortic aneurysm** is often made with x-ray, ultrasound, TEE, CTA, or MRA. Cardiac catheterization and echocardiogram may also be needed for aneurysm of the ascending aorta. Surgery is indicated for both thoracic and abdominal aortic aneurysms when they reach ≥6cm in size or if they show evidence of dissection. Interventions include:

- **Thoracic aortic aneurysm:** Endovascular grafting is routinely done for aneurysms of the descending thoracic aorta. Open surgical repair is required for the ascending aorta or arch, but these surgeries are much more dangerous with higher rates of morbidity and mortality than for abdominal aorta repair. There is a 4% occurrence of paraplegia with thoracic aorta aneurysm repair and increased risk of stroke.
- **Abdominal Aortic aneurysm:** There are two types of surgical repair:
  - Open: An abdominal incision is made with dissection of damaged aorta and a graft is sutured in place. Aortic blood flow must be interrupted with CPB during this procedure.
  - Endovascular: A stent graft is fed through the arteries to line the aorta and exclude the aneurysm.

Complications include myocardial infarction, renal injury can occur, and GI hemorrhage, which may occur up to years after surgery. Endo-leaks can occur with a stent graft, increasing risk of rupture.

VASCULAR INTERVENTION LEADINGS TO COMPLICATIONS
RETROPERITONEAL BLEEDING

Retroperitoneal bleeding may occur as a complication of femoral artery catheterization (such as for PCI procedures) when the artery is perforated or dissected. A large hematoma forms and dissects the artery with bleeding into the retroperitoneum, a life-threatening complication. Factors that increase the risk of perforation include large catheter size, multiple attempts at insertion, long dwell time, inadequate vascular closure, and accidental perforation. Risk of severe hemorrhage is increased with the use of periprocedural anticoagulation and antiplatelet agents. Patients of older age and large size/body weight as well as those with preexisting coagulopathy, hypertension, and renal disease also have increased risk. With bleeding, patients may complain of abdominal, back, or groin pain or swelling, and some may exhibit unexplained hypotension and bradycardia or tachycardia. Diagnosis is confirmed by symptoms and CT. Treatment includes transfusions and surgical repair.

PSEUDOANEURYSMS

Pseudoaneurysm (AKA false aneurysm), which is injury to the inner layers of the arterial wall allowing blood to collect and balloon out between the two outer layers of the arterial wall, results in a thin-walled cavity that is prone to rupture. If all 3 layers of the artery are disrupted, the blood may be contained by surrounding tissue. A pseudoaneurysm may occur with injury to the arterial wall during PCI procedures, especially with femoral catheterization. Blood may leak and pool at the insertion site. Contributing factors include periprocedural anticoagulation, inadequate compression of the insertion site after removal of the catheter, hypertension, and arterial calcifications. Patients may complain of pain about insertion site with a pulsatile mass evident on examination and with a systolic bruit. Diagnosis is per Doppler ultrasound or color flow imaging. Treatment includes watch and wait as small pseudoaneurysms may heal spontaneously, ultrasound-guided compression, ultrasound-guided thrombin injection, or surgical repair.

Monitoring and Diagnostics

ACRONYMS

Acronym	Meaning
CO	Cardiac Output – measures the amount of blood ejected from the heart in one minute.
	Normal range: 4 to 8 L/min.
CI	Cardiac Index – measures cardiac output when compared to the patient's body mass index.
	Normal range: 2.5 to 4 L/min/m2.
SV	Stroke Volume – measures the amount of blood ejected from the heart with each contraction.
	Normal range: 60 to 100 ml/beat.
CVP	Central Venous Pressure, or Right Atrial Pressure (RAP) – measures fluid volume and pressure in the right atrium.
	Normal range: 2 to 6 mmHg.
PAP	Pulmonary Artery Pressure – refers to the amount of resistance in the pulmonary artery. Pulmonary artery diastolic pressure can also be used to determine left ventricular end diastolic pressure (LVEDP).
	Normal range: Pulmonary artery systolic: 15 to 30 mmHg. Pulmonary artery diastolic: 5 to 15 mmHg.
PAWP	Pulmonary Artery Wedge Pressure – reflects left ventricular preload and LVEDP.
	Normal range: 6 to 12 mmHg.
SVR	Systemic Vascular Resistance – refers to left ventricular afterload.
	Normal range: 900 to 1400 dynes/sec/cm-5.

CARDIAC OUTPUT AND CARDIAC INDEX CALCULATIONS

Cardiac output is measured using thermodilution. 10 ml of cold normal saline is injected into the proximal port as quickly as possible. The thermistor on the distal end of the catheter will note the temperature change within the blood, measuring the amount of time it takes for the blood temperature to normalize. When the patient has good cardiac output, it requires a shorter amount of time for the temperature of the blood to normalize. Usually, the cold solution is injected three times, and averaged to obtain a mean cardiac output measure.

The cardiac index is measured by dividing the cardiac output by the patient's body mass index, to account for variability in each patient's body size.

LAB TESTS USED FOR CARDIAC MONITORING AND DIAGNOSTICS

Test	Normal values	Discussion
Aspartate amino-transferase (AST)	Male >50: 10-35 U/L or 0.17-0.6 micro kat/L	Appears in 6-8 hours of MI, peaks at 24-48 hours, and returns to normal in 3 to 4 days. Indicates increased liver enzymes, which often occur with ST-segment elevation STEMI. With acute MI that occurs without shock, the levels may remain fairly stable.
	Female >45: 10-35 U/L or 0.17-0.6 micro kat/L	
Creatine kinase (CK)	Male: 50-204 U/L	Non-specific; found in skeletal muscle, heart muscle, brain and lungs. Increased within 48 hours of acute MI and returns to normal within 3 days.
	Female: 36-160 U/L	
Creatine isoenzyme (CK-MB)	0-4%	Specific to heart muscle. Present within 4 to 6 hours of MI, peaks in 24 hours, and returns to normal in 2 to 3 days. If elevation recurs, it may indicate reinfarction or increased ischemic damage to heart muscle.
Lactate dehydrogenase (LDH)	>Age 43: 90-176 U/L	Increases in 12 hours of MI, peaks at 24 to 48 hours, and returns to normal within 10-14 days. May also increase with diabetes, hemorrhage, liver failure, pulmonary embolism, and shock.
Myoglobin	Male: 28-72 ng/mL or 1.6-4.1 nmol/L	Found in skeletal and heart muscle. Increases in 1-3 hours, peaks at 4 to 12 hours, and resolves within 24 hours.
	Female: 25-58 ng/mL or 1.4-3.3 nmol/L	
Troponin I	<0.05 ng/mL	Appears in 2 to 6 hours, peaks at 15 to 20 hours and returns to normal in 5 to 7 days. Exhibits a second but lower peak at 60 to 80 hour (biphasic).
Troponin T	<0.2 ng/mL.	Increases 2 to 6 hours after MI and stays elevated. Returns to normal in 7 days. (Less specific than troponin I)
Serum creatinine	Male: 0.61-1.21 mg/dL or 54-107 mmol/L	Increased with heart failure, associated with fluid retention and decreased urinary output. Impaired renal function (increased creatinine) correlates with more negative outcomes, including mortality, following MI.
	Female: 0.51-1.11 mg/dL or 45-98 mmol/L	
B-natriuretic peptide (BNP)	<100 pg/mL or ng/L.	>100 pg/mL or ng/L. Non-specific—increased with acute HF, MI, myocarditis, ventricular dysfunction, and left ventricular hypertrophy.

INVASIVE HEMODYNAMIC MONITORING

Hemodynamic monitoring is the monitoring of blood flow, pressures, and volumes. When catheters are placed; the most common sites are the left atrium, right atrium, and pulmonary artery or superior vena cava. Indications for an arterial line include hemodynamic instability, frequent ABG monitoring, placement of IABP, monitoring arterial pressure, and medication administration when venous access cannot be obtained. Arterial pressure is used to help to estimate tissue perfusion in lieu of direct pressure measurement within body organs. Intraarterial blood pressure monitoring is done for systolic, diastolic, and mean arterial pressure (MAP) for conditions that decrease cardiac output, tissue perfusion, or fluid volume.

Normal cardiac output is about 5 liters per minutes at rest for an adult. Under exercise or stress, this volume may multiply 3 or 4 times with concomitant changes in the heart rate (HR) and stroke volume (SV). The basic formula for calculating cardiac output is the heart rate (HR) per minute multiplied by measurement of the stroke volume (SR) (assessed per echocardiogram), which is the amount of blood pumped through the ventricles with each contraction. The stroke volume is controlled by preload, afterload, and contractibility: CO = HR X SV.

PULMONARY ARTERY CATHETER

A pulmonary artery or Swan-Ganz catheter is a device that measures pressure within the right atrium and the pulmonary artery. Pressure in the right atrium is measured using the proximal port, and pressure in the pulmonary artery is measured using the distal port. Because it is not feasible to place a measurement catheter in the left ventricle, pressures are measured indirectly using pressures taken on the right side of the heart. When the balloon in the pulmonary artery is inflated, the pressure in the pulmonary artery gives an indication of left ventricular end-diastolic pressure (LVEDP) and left ventricular preload. A pulmonary artery catheter can also measure the patient's cardiac output, cardiac index, and stroke volume.

INSERTING A PULMONARY ARTERY CATHETER

A pulmonary artery catheter can be inserted at the patient's bedside using sterile technique. The area over the subclavian or jugular vein is numbed using a topical anesthetic. An opening in the skin is created using a large bore needle, and then a Cordis sheath is inserted into the vein. Next, the pulmonary artery catheter is threaded through the vein to the right atrium. The balloon of the pulmonary catheter is then inflated as it is floated to the pulmonary artery. While the pulmonary catheter is being placed, the nurse should monitor the patient's vital signs and the arterial waveform pattern produced as it moves through the heart. The patient should also be monitored for any signs of cardiac ectopy. Once the waveform for the pulmonary artery is visualized, the pulmonary catheter is sutured into place and covered with an occlusive dressing.

CARING FOR A PATIENT WITH A PULMONARY ARTERY CATHETER

The transducer of the pulmonary artery catheter should be kept at the phlebostatic axis to ensure accurate measurements. The catheter dressing should remain clean and intact. The measurements of the pulmonary catheter should be checked regularly to ensure the catheter has not migrated out of position. The patient's arterial waveforms should also be checked to ensure that the catheter is properly placed. After the wedge pressure is obtained the nurse should take care to deflate the balloon, as it will occlude circulation in the pulmonary artery if left inflated. The continued need for a pulmonary artery catheter should be frequently assessed, as it should be discontinued when the patient is hemodynamically stable.

PULMONARY ARTERY WAVEFORM AND ITS REFLECTION OF PULMONARY ARTERY PRESSURE

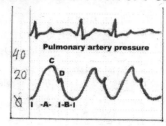

Pulmonary artery pressure (PAP) is measured by a catheter usually fed through the right ventricle to the main pulmonary artery, measuring systolic, diastolic, and mean pressures, with the patient in supine position ≤45° elevation:

- **Normal values:** PA systolic 20-30 mm Hg, diastolic 6-15 mm Hg. Postoperative rates should be <25 mm Hg. PAP is usually about 25-34% the systemic blood pressure rate. Oxygen saturation is usually about 80%.
- **Increased pressure** may indicate pulmonary obstruction or embolus, left to right shunt, left ventricular failure, pulmonary hypertension, or mitral stenosis, pneumothorax, lung/alveolar hypoplasia, hyperviscosity of blood, or increased left atrial pressure.
- **Decreased pressure** may indicate a decrease in intravascular volume or cardiac output, or obstruction of pulmonary blood flow. **On the diagram, A** represents systole; **B**, diastole; **C**, peak systole; and **D** (dicrotic notch), closure of pulmonic valve. The pulmonary artery catheter may have a balloon that can be inflated in the pulmonary artery to provide a measurement of pulmonary artery/capillary wedge pressure (PAWP/PCWP) to evaluate pulmonary hypertension, left ventricular failure, and mitral stenosis: Normal values 4-12 mm Hg. Increased pressure may indicate left ventricular failure, mitral insufficiency, or mitral stenosis.

COMPLICATIONS

While the patient has a pulmonary artery catheter, they are at an increased risk for cardiac arrhythmias from irritation to the heart caused by the catheter. The patient is also at risk for rupture of the pulmonary artery as a result of insertion or migration of the pulmonary artery catheter. Patients with a pulmonary artery catheter are also at risk for damage to the tricuspid or pulmonary valves, or developing endocarditis.

While the pulmonary artery catheter is in place, the patient should also be closely monitored for signs and symptoms of infection, including redness or purulent drainage at the catheter insertion site. Their heart rhythm and rate should also be closely monitored.

CENTRAL VENOUS PRESSURE MEASUREMENT, VALUES, AND INDICATIONS

Central venous pressure (CVP), the pressure in the right atrium or vena cava, is used to assess function of the right ventricles, preload, and flow of venous blood to the heart. Central lines may be placed into the internal jugular vein (right preferred), subclavian vein, or femoral vein (usually avoided) to help determine hemodynamic therapy. Indications include hypovolemic shock, postoperative monitoring, and confirmation of right-sided heart failure. CVP is no longer used to determine fluid replacement needs. CVP can be monitored manually with a manometer or electronically with a transducer that displays a continuous waveform on a monitor. Normal pressure ranges from 2-6 mm Hg but may be elevated after cardiac surgery to 6-8 mm Hg. Incorrect catheter placement or malfunctioning can affect readings.

- **Increased CVP** is related to overload of intravascular volume caused by decreased function, hypertrophy, or failure of the right ventricle; increased right ventricular afterload, tricuspid valve stenosis, regurgitation, or thrombus obstruction; or shunt from left ventricle to right atrium. It can also be caused by arrhythmias or cardiac tamponade and fluid overload.
- **Decreased CVP** is related to low intravascular volume, decreased preload, vasodilation, and distributive shock.

PLACEMENT OF ECG LEADS FOR A FIVE LEAD SYSTEM

Placement of the ECG leads is determined by color. The right arm (RA) lead (white) is placed below the patient's right clavicle. The left arm (LA) lead (black) should be placed below the patient's left clavicle. The right leg (RL) lead (green) is placed on the right side of the patient's lower abdomen. The left leg (LL) lead (red) is placed on the left side of the patient's lower abdomen. The C lead (brown) is placed on the right side of the sternal border. A mnemonic for remembering the positioning of the leads is "White is right, snow over grass, smoke over fire, and brown is in the middle."

PLACEMENT OF 12-LEAD ECG LEADS

The **electrocardiogram** provides a graphic representation of the electrical activity of the heart. It is indicated for chest pain, dyspnea, syncope, acute coronary syndrome, pulmonary embolism, and possible MI. The standard 12-lead ECG gives a picture of electrical activity from 12 perspectives through placement of 10 body leads:

- 4 limb leads are placed distally on the wrists and ankles (but may be placed more proximally if necessary).
- Precordial leads:
  - V1: right sternal border at 4th intercostal space.
  - V2: left sternal border at 4th intercostal space.
  - V3: Midway between V2 and V4.
  - V4: Left midclavicular line at 5th intercostal space.
  - V5: Horizontal to V4 at left anterior axillary line.
  - V6: Horizontal to V5 at left midaxillary line.
- In some cases, additional leads may be used:
  - Right-sided leads are placed on the right in a mirror image of the left leads, usually to diagnose right ventricular infarction through ST elevation.

CARDIAC MONITORING

There are a number of indications for placing a patient on cardiac monitoring. The patient should be placed on cardiac monitoring to check cardiac medication efficacy, or when adjusting dosages of cardiac medications. The patient should also be placed on a monitor following any cardiac procedures, such as cardiac catheterization, cardiac surgery, pacemaker placement, or an ablation. The patient should receive cardiac monitoring if they have any electrolyte imbalances that might affect heart rate or rhythm. Cardiac monitoring is also indicated if the patient has symptoms such as shortness of breath, chest pain, palpitations, or dizziness. Finally, the patient should be monitored if they have a history of, or currently have, any tachyarrhythmias, bradyarrhythmias, or ECG changes.

CONTINUOUS ST SEGMENT MONITORING

Continuous ST segment monitoring is indicated to assess transient myocardial ischemia for patients with:

- Acute coronary syndrome.
- Unstable angina.
- Myocardial infarction.

ST segment elevation is found when ischemia is transmural, often indicating a myocardial infarction. ST elevation generally indicates the need for immediate intervention to improve blood flow to the heart. ST depression, on the other hand, is found with myocardial ischemia that is subendocardial and usually associated with coronary artery insufficiency. With ST depression, the oxygen supply to the heart is inadequate for needs, such as may occur when patients exercise or experience tachycardia. If the ST change is ≥2mm for 15 minutes, a 12-lead ECG should be taken to confirm elevation or depression. If ST segment changes are noted, the nurse should make sure that the patient is correctly positioned (supine, <45° head elevation) and that leads are in intact and positioned correctly to ensure that readings are accurate. In addition to ischemia, ST changes may be caused by intermittent RBBB, LBBB, dysrhythmias, pericarditis, digoxin (depression) myocardial contusion, and ventricular paced rhythms.

CONTINUOUS QT INTERVAL MONITORING

Continuous QT interval monitoring measures from the QRS complex (depolarization) to the end of the T wave (repolarization). Indications (AHA recommendations) include patients that are:

- Newly diagnosed with bradyarrhythmia.
- Receiving anti-arrhythmic drugs or other drugs associated with torsade de pointes (a life-threatening dysrhythmia).
- Overdosing on agents or receiving antipsychotics or drugs that may cause arrhythmias.
- With electrolyte imbalances (hypokalemia, hypomagnesemia) that may cause arrhythmias.
- With acute neurological events, such as stroke.

The normal QT interval is greater than 460 ms in females and greater than 440 ms in male. QT interval value greater than 500 ms increases risk of torsades de pointes. If the QT interval extends greater than half the RR, it is prolonged. Long QT syndrome occurs when depolarization and repolarization is prolonged between beats and can result in torsades de points or VT. Long QT syndrome may be a genetic condition or may be acquired and associated with electrolyte imbalances, some medications (antidepressants, diuretics, antibiotics), and some conditions (anorexia nervosa).

IMPROVING AN ECG TRACING

If there is too much artifact to obtain a good ECG tracing, there are a number of steps that can be taken to improve the output. Make sure the skin beneath the electrodes is clean and free of hair. If necessary, shave the skin where the leads will be placed to ensure good contact and adherence. Check the pads to make sure the electrode gel has not dried. Also, check to make sure the electrode is pressed firmly against the skin. If necessary, remove the electrodes and readjust the lead placement to ensure a good tracing. If problems continue, check the ECG wires to make sure they are properly connected.

PROPER DOCUMENTATION OF ECG

Documentation for cardiac monitoring should be completed, at a minimum, as follows: 1) once on admission, 2) once each shift, and 3) at the time of any ECG changes. When recordkeeping, the patient's heart rate and rhythm should be recorded and the PR, QRS and QT intervals should be measured using calipers and also recorded. Further, an ECG strip should be placed on the patient's chart at each of the aforementioned times, to help in pinpointing the time of any ECG changes. If any symptomatic ECG changes occur, the physician should be notified, and the patient should be treated as ordered.

TRANSESOPHAGEAL ECHOCARDIOGRAM PROCEDURE

The **transesophageal echocardiogram** procedure is as follows:

- The back of the patient's throat is sprayed (or patient asked to gargle) with an anesthetic agent to numb the back of the throat and decrease the gag reflex.
- The patient receives conscious sedation so that the patient is relaxed but can follow directions and is placed on left side with left arm behind back.
- A mouthguard is placed inside the patient's mouth to prevent the patient from biting the physician's finger or the probe.
- The patient is asked to take deep slow breaths in order to relax the esophagus.
- The patient is asked to tuck the chin to the chest and open the mouth.
- The flexible ultrasound probe is slowly inserted through the mouthguard while the patient swallows.
- The probe is advanced into the esophagus about 14 to 18 inches.
- Images are viewed on the video screen and recorded for 15 to 30 minutes, with the probe occasionally repositioned to improve the images.
- Once the echocardiogram is completed, the probe is pulled out slowly and mouthguard removed.

TRANSTHORACIC ECHOCARDIOGRAM PROCEDURE

The **transthoracic echocardiogram** is a non-invasive ultrasound imaging of the heart obtained through a transducer applied to the skin. No special preparation is needed for the test. **Procedure**:

- The patient is asked to disrobe above the waist and put on a gown that opens in the front to allow access to the chest.
- Leads for a 3-lead ECG are applied in order to monitor heart function.
- Lights are dimmed to reduce glare on the video monitor.
- The patient is initially in supine position but is then positioned on the left side on the examining table and may be asked periodically to change position.
- Water soluble gel is applied to the tip (probe) of the transducer and the probe placed firmly against the skin.
- The probe is moved about the chest and placed in different positions in order to record the size, shape, and functions of the heart and take different views of the heart.
- The length of the procedure varies but usually is about 30 to 45 minutes, including time preparing and positioning patient.
- Once the echocardiogram is completed, the ECG leads are removed and the soluble gel wiped from the skin.
- The patient redresses and requires no further post-echo treatment or monitoring.

TESTS INVOLVED IN A BASIC METABOLIC PANEL

A basic metabolic panel (BMP) is a collection of seven tests that are typically obtained while a patient is in the intensive care unit. The tests include four electrolyte measures, specifically: sodium, potassium, chloride, and bicarbonate. Further, blood urea nitrogen (BUN) and creatinine levels are also obtained through a BMP. These two levels provide an indication of the patient's kidney function status. Finally, a blood glucose is also included in a BMP. A BMP is typically drawn on a daily basis during an ICU stay. However, the BMP may be done more often, depending upon the patient's diagnosis and electrolyte status.

TESTS INVOLVED IN A COMPREHENSIVE METABOLIC PANEL

A comprehensive metabolic panel (CMP) consists of the seven tests found in the basic metabolic panel, as well as seven additional tests. If possible, the patient should fast for ten to twelve hours prior to blood for this metabolic panel being drawn. The comprehensive metabolic panel includes testing for an additional electrolyte, calcium. Also included in a CMP are two protein tests that help to diagnose liver or kidney disorders, specifically: human serum albumin and the total serum protein. Four liver function tests are also included, specifically: alkaline phosphatase, alanine amino transferase, aspartate amino transferase, and bilirubin.

BASIC ASPECTS OF A COMPLETE BLOOD COUNT

A complete blood count (CBC) is a common test performed while a patient is in a critical care unit. It measures the patient's red and white blood cell counts, and may provide a "differential" description of the types of white blood cells noted. A CBC also includes the amount of hemoglobin in the blood. Hematocrit (the ratio of red blood cells compared to the total volume of blood) is also included in a CBC. Mean corpuscular volume (MCV) measures the size of red blood cells. Mean corpuscular hematocrit (MCH) calculates the amount of oxygen-carrying hemoglobin in each red blood cell. Mean corpuscular hemoglobin concentration (MCHC) measures the average amount of hemoglobin in each red blood cell. Red blood cell distribution width (RDW) measures the variation in sizes of the red blood cells (as immature red cells tend to be larger). Finally, the platelet count indicates the patient's platelet level.

IMPLICATIONS OF AN ABNORMAL COMPLETE BLOOD COUNT

An elevated white blood cell (WBC) count indicates an infection. A change in the WBC differential can indicate the type and progression of the infection. The WBC count may be decreased in cases of autoimmune diseases or leukemia. A low red blood cell (RBC) count indicates anemia. An elevated RBC may indicate dehydration. Hemoglobin (HGB) and hematocrit (HCT) results mirror RBC count. If the mean corpuscular volume (MCV) is elevated, it indicates a vitamin B12 or folate deficiency. The MCV is decreased in iron deficiency. Mean corpuscular hemoglobin (MCH) and mean corpuscular hemoglobin concentration (MCHC) results should mirror the MCV results. The patient's platelet count may be decreased if the patient is bleeding.

PT, INR, AND aPTT BLOOD TESTS

Prothrombin Time (PT) is a test that measures the amount of time it takes for a patient's blood plasma to clot. The International Normalized Ratio (INR) is a measure derived from a patient's prothrombin time (the ratio of the patient's PT to a standardized PT rate. PT and INR tests are most commonly ordered to check the effectiveness of an anticoagulation therapy regimen, usually determining a proper Coumadin dosage. This may be done daily, on an inpatient basis. PT and INR tests can also be obtained to assess a patient's liver function. Elevated PT and INR rates, without the presence of anticoagulation therapy, may indicate liver damage. In such situations, PT and INR rates may be checked as often as every 4 hours to monitor the progression of liver failure.

An activated partial thromboplastin time (aPTT) is typically drawn to assess the efficacy of a heparin dosage. However, an elevated aPTT without the presence of heparin may indicate lupus or certain types of genetic clotting disorders.

RESULTS OF PT, APTT, AND INR TESTING

Coagulation studies are performed when a patient is receiving an anticoagulation medication to ensure a proper therapeutic dosage. Prothrombin time (PT) and the international normalized ratio (INR) both measure the extrinsic pathway of anticoagulation. The normal range for a PT result is between 13 and 17 seconds. The normal range for the INR is between 0.8 and 1.2. For anticoagulation therapy to be deemed successful, the PT result obtained should be two to three times the patient's baseline PT rate.

An activated partial thromboplastin time (aPTT) measures the effectiveness of both the extrinsic and intrinsic clotting pathway. It is typically used to monitor the effectiveness of heparin therapy. The typical range for an aPTT result is 20 to 36 seconds.

CARDIAC STRESS TESTING

The **cardiac stress test** is used to diagnose and/or evaluate coronary artery disease, angina, functional capacity of heart, effectiveness of medication, dysrhythmias, and attainment of physical fitness goals. Normal coronary arteries dilate to 4 times the resting diameter when under stress, so testing to determine if there is compromised blood flow is more accurate under exercise conditions:

- **Exercise stress test:** Usually done with the person walking on a treadmill or pedaling a stationary bicycle. The most common procedure is the Bruce protocol in which the speed and grade of the treadmill increases every 3 minutes. The goal is to increase the heart rate to 80-90% of predicted heart rate for age and gender. During testing, the heart is monitored with an ECG, and BP and oxygen saturation are monitored as well.
- **Pharmacologic stress test:** Used for those unable to tolerate the exercise test or are at high risk of coronary artery heart disease and to assess presurgical risks. An agent (dobutamine, adenosine, dipyridamole) is administered to slowly increase the heart rate, and the effects monitored with ECG, echocardiogram and/or radionuclide imaging. Cardiolite (a radioactive tracer) may be administered.

PRE- AND POST-PROCEDURE MANAGEMENT

Cardiac stress testing:

- **Pre-procedure management:** Outpatients should be provided written instructions. Patients should avoid any products (foods, drinks, medications) that contain caffeine for 24 hours prior to the exam because of their stimulating effect. Additionally, patients are usually advised to stop beta blockers 48 hours before test and calcium channel blockers 24 hours before. If having the myocardial infusion SPECT test, the patient should be questioned about claustrophobia because some feel excessively constrained by the camera. Patients should avoid food or drink (except for water) for at 3-6 hours prior to the test. VS should be assessed before the patient begins the test. Allergies (for pharmacologic testing) should be assessed.
- **Post-procedure management:** The patient's vital signs should be monitored and the physician notified of any emergent symptoms, such as severe chest pain or dysrhythmias. Patients can generally resume eating and drinking and taking medications following the test.

Assistive Devices

INTRA-AORTIC BALLOON PUMP
IMPROVEMENT OF CARDIAC FUNCTION

The intra-aortic balloon pump (IABP) rests in the patient's descending aorta. The machine console coordinates the inflation of the balloon with the patient's cardiac cycle, inflating the balloon at the start of diastole, and deflating the balloon at the beginning systole. As the balloon inflates, arterial perfusion pressure increases. Peripheral perfusion improves, as does coronary artery perfusion. Prior to systole, the balloon will deflate, improving the ejection fraction by drawing blood into the aorta by creating a vacuum effect. In this way, cardiac workload is reduced while contractility and cardiac output is improved by as much as 40%.

INDICATIONS

The primary indication for an intra-aortic balloon pump (IABP) is hypoperfusion secondary to cardiogenic shock. Because the heart is impaired, an IABP is placed to improve cardiac output and to maintain the patient's blood pressure. Other indications for the placement of an IABP include left ventricular impairment (typically with an ejection fraction less than 30%), and the treatment of complications following a percutaneous coronary intervention.

The IABP is a polyethylene balloon mounted on a catheter, and is typically inserted into the femoral artery through a sheath. The balloon is moved upward into the artery until it is placed below the aortic arch and above the renal arteries. Because placement of an IABP is done in a cardiac cath lab, placement is confirmed under fluoroscopy.

COMPLICATIONS

The most common complication related to intra-aortic balloon pump (IABP) placement is limb ischemia. This may occur as a result of thromboembolism (usually secondary to the presence of atherosclerosis), balloon displacement, or injury to the artery during IABP placement. The patient is also at risk for bleeding secondary to insertion of the IABP within the femoral artery (and related thrombolytic therapy), or as a result of aortic dissection. If the patient is not given anticoagulation therapy, a thromboembolic disorder may develop secondary to thrombus formation on the balloon. The patient's white blood cell count should be monitored for signs of infection related to IABP placement. Though it is rare, the patient may develop an air embolism if the balloon ruptures.

CARING FOR A PATIENT WITH AN INTRA-AORTIC BALLOON PUMP

The patient's vital signs should be closely monitored to ensure hemodynamic stability. The intra-aortic balloon pump (IABP) console settings and sequencing should be checked regularly to ensure the balloon is inflating at the proper time in the cardiac cycle. Frequent pain assessments should also be performed, and any pain should be treated appropriately. Vascular assessments should be completed regularly to ensure the balloon is not occluding circulation to the extremities. The insertion site in the femoral artery should also be closely monitored to ensure that no complications occur at the site, such as hematoma or pseudoaneurysm. The patient's urinary output should also be monitored, as oliguria may indicate the balloon is occluding the renal arteries. The IABP catheter tubing should be regularly checked for the presence of any blood, as this indicates rupture of the balloon.

WEANING INTRA-AORTIC BALLOON PUMP DEPENDENCE

It is appropriate to begin weaning the patient away from the intra-aortic balloon pump (IABP) when the patient is deemed hemodynamically stable. A patient is considered stable when they can maintain a mean arterial blood pressure greater than 65 mmHg without vasopressors, and maintain a cardiac index greater than 2.5 L/min/m². The IABP can be weaned by decreasing balloon volume or by decreasing the rate of augmentation. The rate of augmentation is set to one augmentation for every 2 heartbeats (1:2). If the patient remains hemodynamically stable, the rate of augmentation is decreased to one augmentation for every three heart beats (1:3). If the patient continues to remains hemodynamically stable for six hours on 1:3, it is considered safe to remove the IABP. Any thrombolytic therapy is discontinued at least 6 hours prior to removal of the IABP to decrease the risk of bleeding as the catheter is removed.

Cardiac and Vascular Procedures

CAROTID ANGIOGRAPHY INDICATIONS AND PROCEDURE DETAILS

Carotid angiography is indicated to confirm carotid stenosis when a bruit is heard or when the patient experiences TIE, when stroke risk needs to be assessed, and to determine the need for further interventions, such as CEA or carotid stent. Contraindications to carotid angiography include complete carotid occlusion, stenosis of the artery with thick calcifications, and history of severe stroke, advanced dementia, cerebral hemorrhage, and brain tumor. Carotid angiography is generally carried out in the cardiac cath lab. Procedure:

- Patient fasts for 6 hours except for sips of water to take medications. Anticoagulants are held as determined by physician and diabetic medications are withheld the morning of the examination.
- Patient is positioned on table in supine position.
- Patient receives sedative, often conscious sedation.
- After a local anesthetic is applied, the catheter is inserted into either the radial or femoral artery and passed to the carotid artery, dye injected, and images obtained.
- Once the catheter is removed, pressure is applied to the site, the site monitored for signs of bleeding or other complications.

Possible **complications** include stroke, MI, hemorrhage, thrombus formation, carotid occlusion, and death.

CAROTID ARTERY STENTING

INDICATIONS

Carotid artery stenting is a minimally invasive procedure to place a stent in a carotid artery in order to improve blood flow to the brain and reduce the risk of stroke. Indications include:

- Presence of symptoms with ≥70% stenosis.
- Lack of symptoms but >60% stenosis.
- Presence of symptoms with 50 to 69% stenosis.

Patients may also be considered for stenting if they are not candidates for CEA, had previous surgery on the same side of the neck, received radiotherapy of the neck, and had injury to the contralateral vocal cord. Contraindications to carotid artery stenting are similar to those of carotid angiography and include complete carotid occlusion, stenosis of the artery with thick calcifications (unstable plaques), and history of severe stroke, advanced dementia, cerebral hemorrhage, and brain tumor. Complications include stroke, recurrence of arterial stenosis, hyperperfusion syndrome post-procedure (intracranial hemorrhage, seizures, headache).

PROCEDURE

Carotid artery stenting procedure:

- Initial preparation and positioning is similar to that for carotid angiography. In most cases, patients are advised to take aspirin and clopidogrel for a week prior to the position to decrease the risk of thrombosis. Additionally, many patients take a statin for a few weeks before the procedure. For those already on anticoagulant therapy, the physician will guide dosage.
- The patient is placed in supine position with neck slightly extended and administered sedation (conscious sedation most common) and a local anesthetic administered to insertion site (usually the femoral artery).
- The catheter with an angioplasty balloon is inserted through the artery and advanced to the carotid artery and the balloon inflated to increase lumen size. An embolic protection device may be inserted. The balloon is deflated and withdrawn.
- A second catheter with a compressed stent is threaded to the target area.
- The stent is threaded through the occluded area, released, and expanded to open the artery and the catheter removed.
- The stent may be further expanded with a balloon catheter.
- The catheters and embolic protective device rare removed, compression applied to insertion site, and the patient monitored for bleeding, stroke or other complications.

CATHETER-DIRECTED THROMBOLYSIS

INDICATIONS

Catheter-directed thrombolysis is a minimally-invasive procedure used to dissolve thrombi by feeding a catheter through the common femoral artery to the site of occlusion and administration of a thrombolytic agent directly into the thrombus in order to improve blood flow and reduce symptoms. Fluoroscopy and a video monitor are used to ensure proper placement of the catheter and thrombolytic agent. Indications for catheter-directed thrombolysis include: acute ischemia of a limb, thrombosis associated with severe atherosclerosis, DVT, clotted dialysis fistula/graft, portal vein thrombosis, pulmonary embolus, and other emboli. Absolute contraindications to catheter-directed thrombolysis include: TIE or stroke within the previous 2 months, active bleeding or recent GI bleeding, history of neurological surgery, or intracranial trauma in the previous 3 months. Relative contraindications include a history of CPR or major surgery or trauma in the previous 10 days, hypertension >180/>110, history of recent ophthalmic surgery, and intracranial tumor.

PROCEDURE

Catheter-directed thrombolysis procedure:

- Patient stops taking anticoagulants, ASA, or NSAIDS a few days prior to the procedure.
- Patient is NPO for at least 6 hours prior to the procedure.
- Patient placed in supine position on the table and connected to a cardiac monitor.
- IV line inserted to provide conscious sedation (or general anesthesia administered).
- The skin at insertion site (usually the femoral artery) prepped, patient draped, and local anesthetic administered.
- Catheter inserted and contrast dye injected and images taken to ensure accurate placement of the catheter.
- Thrombolytic agent injected into the clot or a mechanical device used to break up the thrombus or suction it from the vessel.

- Catheter may be left in place for a few hours to 2 to 3 days and attached to a pump that delivers the thrombolytic agent at a specific rate until the clot dissolves.
- After catheter removal, compression applied to the site to prevent bleeding and the patient carefully monitored for complications, such as retroperitoneal hemorrhage, stroke, intracranial hemorrhage, or infection.

ENDOVASCULAR GRAFTS

INDICATIONS

Endovascular grafting (AKA endovascular stent grafts or endovascular aneurysm repair [EVAR]) is a minimally-invasive procedure primarily used to treat thoracic or abdominal aortic aneurysms but can also be used on other aneurysms. During the procedure, an expandable stent graft (a fabric tube with wire mesh supports) attached to a catheter is inserted into the aorta, positioned at the aneurysm, and expanded to provide a secure open vessel and then the catheter removed. The graft extends both above and below the aneurysm to ensure blood flows only through the stent graft. Indications include:

- Aneurysm ≥5 cm in diameter.
- Dissecting aneurysm in risk of rupture.
- Rapidly growing aneurysm (greater than 1 cm/yr).
- Aneurysm with symptoms, such as severe pain, or chronic pain in back or abdomen.

Some patients are not candidates for endovascular graft because of the location of condition of the artery or preexisting conditions, such as Marfan disease.

PROCEDURE

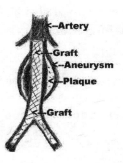

Endovascular graft procedure:

- Patient generally stops taking anticoagulants, ASA, or NSAIDS a few days prior to the procedure.
- Patient placed in supine position, prepped and draped, IV inserted, and cardiac monitoring carried out.
- Anesthesia varies but may include local with conscious sedation, general anesthesia, or spinal anesthesia.
- A spinal drainage catheter may be placed.
- Both right and left femoral arteries may be cannulated, contrast dye injected, and images taken to ensure accurate placement of catheters, and arch arteriogram for thoracic repair.
- The catheter with the graft is threaded to the aneurysm, positioned under fluoroscopy, and the stent released so that it expands above and below the aneurysm to prevent blood flow around the graft. In some cases, more than one graft is necessary.
- The catheter is removed and compression applied to insertion sites to prevent bleeding.

Complications include paralysis, infection, bleeding about the graft (endoleak), migration of the stent, kidney damage, and arterial occlusion. In some cases, a delayed rupture may still occur with endoleak.

PERCUTANEOUS CORONARY INTERVENTION

A percutaneous coronary intervention (PCI) is done during a cardiac catheterization to treat occluded coronary arteries. The most common procedure performed during a PCI is a percutaneous transluminal coronary angioplasty (PTCA). During PTCA, a small balloon is inflated within the coronary artery, pushing atherosclerotic plaque against the walls of the artery and opening the vessel. During a PTCA, a mesh wire tube, known as a stent, may be placed. When the angioplasty balloon is inflated, the stent opens; it remains open to keep the coronary artery expanded.

Conversely, atherosclerotic plaque may be removed using a cutting balloon (directional coronary atherectomy), various other catheter-introduced cutting devices (e.g., rotational atherectomy and extraction atherectomy), or lasers. Another technique is to use radioactivity to prevent re-stenosis, referred to as intravascular brachytherapy (IVBT).

CARDIAC CATHETERIZATION AND PERCUTANEOUS CORONARY INTERVENTION

A percutaneous coronary intervention (PCI) is indicated to treat symptoms of coronary artery disease. It should be considered for patients who experience angina or ECG changes during a stress test. PCI may be indicated if medical management is unsuccessful in patients with chest pain, dyspnea, or heart failure. A cardiac catheterization should also be considered for investigational purposes, in cases of cardiomegaly, congestive heart failure, valvular heart disease, and in evaluation of the need for heart transplantation.

An emergent cardiac catheterization and PCI should also be considered for patients showing signs and symptoms of ST elevation myocardial infarction.

LEFT VS. RIGHT-SIDED CARDIAC CATHETERIZATION

Cardiac catheterization is a minimally-invasive procedure in which a catheter is inserted into the femoral or radial artery and threaded into the right or left side of the heart in order to diagnose, treat, or monitor cardiac conditions. Cardiac catheterization is fluoroscopy guided, and contrast dye is injected for angiography.

Cardiac catheterization	Right heart
Indications	Identify abnormal blood flow.
	Monitor cardiac and pulmonary pressures. Diagnose/treat cardiac tamponade, valve disease, HF, pulmonary hypertension, shock, congenital heart defects, and cardiomyopathy. Monitor damage and treatment for MI. Evaluate CO, LV filling pressure, PAWP, and oxygen saturation. Biopsy heart transplants.
Risks	Pneumothorax, cardiac tamponade, infection, embolism, hypotension, rupture of pulmonary artery, air embolism, dysrhythmias (VT).

TESTS PRIOR TO CARDIAC CATHETERIZATION

Prior to cardiac catheterization, a complete physical examination and past medical history intake is obtained from the patient. An electrocardiogram and chest X-ray is performed. Relevant blood work should include: 1) a complete blood count to rule out a low hemoglobin level, indicating reduced oxygen-carrying capacity, or a low platelet count, which would indicate an increased risk for bleeding; and, 2) a complete metabolic panel should be obtained to check for electrolyte imbalances. Except in cases of emergency, therapy for any electrolyte imbalances should be initiated prior to cardiac catheterization. Female patients should also receive a pregnancy test prior to cardiac catheterization, as X-rays are harmful to fetal development.

NURSING CONSIDERATIONS

Prior to the procedure, the patient and family should be informed of the purpose of the cardiac catheterization and the risks and benefits involved. The patient should be informed about what to expect during the procedure itself. It is also important to ascertain if the patient has any known allergies to contrast dye, strawberries, or shellfish, as allergies to these items will require pre-procedural medication with antihistamines and corticosteroids to prevent a reaction to the contrast dye used during the cardiac catheterization.

The patient should be NPO (fasting) for 4-6 hours prior to the procedure. Subcutaneous insulin dosages should be adjusted to take into account the patient's NPO status. Oral hypoglycemic agents such as metformin should be held for 24 to 48 hours prior to and after a cardiac catheterization as it may have nephrotoxic effects in conjunction with the contrast dye. Anticoagulation therapy should be held for 48 to 72 hours prior to the procedure to decrease risk of bleeding.

INTERVENTION PROCEDURE

The patient is brought to the cardiac catheterization lab and placed on continuous cardiac monitoring. The area over the femoral artery is clipped and cleansed with alcohol. The area over the femoral artery is then numbed using a local anesthetic. The femoral artery is accessed using an introducer needle, and a sheath is slid over the needle to provide continuous access into the artery. A guide-wire is then inserted into the sheath, and threaded up the artery and into the heart. Using contrast dye and real-time x-ray imaging, the coronary arteries are explored for evidence of any occlusions. If an occlusion is located, an angioplasty balloon is slid over the guide wire, and guided to the occlusion site. In cases of balloon angioplasty, a balloon is inflated, pushing the atherosclerotic plaque aside and opening up the coronary artery. If necessary, a stent may be placed over the lesion to prevent reocclusion of the artery. In cases of PCI atherectomy procedures, catheter-introduced cutting devices are used to trim, suction, and remove the identified plaque deposits.

ELEVATED ACTIVATED CLOTTING TIME

Activated clotting time (ACT) measures the amount of time it takes for platelets to aggregate. Prior to a cardiac catheterization, the patient is given a bolus of heparin – typically 100 to 150 units/kg in order to elevate the patient's ACT. This is done to prevent clots from forming on the sheath or within the coronary artery. The patient's ACT is checked every 5 to 10 minutes during the cardiac catheterization, and additional heparin boluses may be administered to maintain an ACT level greater than 300 seconds.

Because the patient's clotting time remains elevated immediately after the procedure, some doctors prefer to wait until the patient's ACT normalizes before removing the femoral artery sheath. The sheath is may be left in the femoral artery, with the patient on strict bed rest, until their ACT is between 75 and 90 seconds.

CARDIAC CATHETERIZATION CLOSURE DEVICES

After the femoral artery sheath is removed, manual pressure may be applied to achieve hemostasis at the insertion site. Other noninvasive methods to apply necessary pressure on the site include the FemoStop or a C-clamp. While the pressure device is in place, the patient will be required to stay on strict bed rest. Bed rest may continue for up to 12 hours after hemostasis has been achieved, depending on facility policy and the patient's risk factors for bleeding.

Invasive closure devices are typically placed by the physician based upon individual preference. Angio-Seal and VasoSeal are collagen plug devices that are inserted into the femoral artery to prevent bleeding. A Perclose is a suture that is placed directly into the artery to prevent bleeding. A SyvekPatch is a dressing that is placed over the insertion site to encourage hemostasis. The period of bed rest required with each of these closure devices is dependent upon specific manufacturer guidelines, but is typically less than that of compression devices.

SYMPTOMS

The patient may experience a pinching and burning sensation at the insertion site of the local anesthetic. The patient may also experience a "flushing" sensation as the contrast dye is injected into the coronary arteries. There is a risk for nausea, vomiting, and cardiac palpitations as a result of injection of the contrast dye. Further, because they must lie still for an extended period of time, some patients may complain of back pain or stiffness. Patients with chronic back pain may be particularly susceptible to this discomfort. The patient may also have a brief moment of chest pain while the angioplasty balloon is inflated. After the balloon is deflated, a brief episode of cardiac dysrhythmias may occur as a result of the restoration of blood flow to ischemic cardiac tissues.

INTERVENTION COMPLICATIONS

The most common risk involved in cardiac catheterization is bleeding at the catheter insertion site. This is partly due to the anticoagulation medications that are given during cardiac catheterization. The patient may also experience bruising or development of a hematoma at the insertion site. There is also a risk for an allergic reaction to the contrast dye. As a result of exposure to contrast dye, the patient is also at risk for subsequent kidney injury.

Though rare, perforation of the arterial wall can occur during the cardiac catheterization. The patient is also at risk for retroperitoneal bleed, and hypovolemia or hypotension. The most serious complications related to a cardiac catheterization are stroke as a result of a dislodged embolus, myocardial infarction, aortic dissection, or death.

NURSING CONSIDERATIONS

After a cardiac catheterization, the patient should stay on strict bed rest for a minimum of one hour, and potentially longer depending upon the type of closure device used. During that time, the patient should be closely monitored for bleeding, hematoma development, or the presence of a bruit at the sheath insertion site. Vital signs should be carefully monitored -- typically every 15 minutes for an hour, every 30 minutes for 2 hours, and then every hour for 4 hours. The patient can resume activity as tolerated within six hours after the PCI. The patient should be orally hydrated to help flush the contrast dye from their blood stream.

After the cardiac catheterization, the patient's BUN and creatinine should be checked to monitor for renal injury as a result of the contrast dye. A complete blood count should be obtained immediately after the procedure and again six hours afterward to monitor for any signs of bleeding. Any complaints of flank or lower back pain should be promptly investigated, as they may result from a retroperitoneal bleed.

MEDICATIONS USED IN CONJUNCTION WITH CARDIAC CATHETERIZATION

To decrease the risk of clot formation at the insertion site or within the stent, the patient is typically started on an antiplatelet agent to prevent platelet aggregation. The most common medication used for this purpose is a glycoprotein IIb/IIIa inhibitor such as Integrilin. The patient will also receive unfractionated heparin to elevate the activated clotting time (ACT) and prevent platelet aggregation during the cardiac catheterization. Antiplatelet medications such as Aspirin and Clopidogrel are typically prescribed after the cardiac catheterization to prevent platelet aggregation on and around the stent.

Nitrates are given prior to cardiac catheterization to prevent angina, and after the procedure to treat chest pain related to vasospasm. Beta-blockers and ACE inhibitors may be prescribed after a myocardial infarction to decrease cardiac workload by lowering the heart rate and blood pressure. Ongoing lipid lowering agents may be prescribed to decrease the buildup of atherosclerotic plaque over time.

PERCUTANEOUS CORONARY INTERVENTION

Percutaneous coronary intervention (PCI) (AKA angioplasty with stent) is a minimally-invasive procedure in which a stent is placed in a coronary artery to improve blood flow in arteries blocked by atherosclerotic plaques. Indications include acute STEMI, non-ST-elevation ACS, angina (stable or unstable), or abnormal stress test findings. Contraindications include long-term treatment with antiplatelet medications and severe life-threatening comorbidities. A relative contraindication is coronary arteries of less than 1.5 mm diameter. **Procedure**:

- Patient NPO for at least 6 hours prior to procedure and may have medications adjusted prior to procedure.
- Patient positioned supine on table, IV started, and cardiac monitoring.
- Patient prepped and draped.
- Patient administered conscious sedation and local anesthetic to insertion site (usually femoral or radial).
- Catheter inserted and threaded to the heart and coronary arteries, contrast dye injected, images taken.
- The balloon catheter positioned at the occluded area and balloon inflated and deflated a number of times.
- The stent positioned and expanded to provide an open lumen for blood flow.
- Catheter removed and pressure applied to insertion site.
- Patient monitored for complications, which can include MI, stroke, pulmonary embolism, and myocardial ischemia from distal embolus.

PERIPHERAL ANGIOGRAPHY AND THE STENTING PROCEDURE

Peripheral angiography is a form of imaging to evaluate peripheral circulation and identify areas of blockage or abnormalities in the arteries of the lower extremities or (in rare occasions) the upper extremities. The procedure involves insertion of a catheter into the femoral artery (most common) or the radial or brachial artery and injection of iodine-based contrast medium to outline the arteries for imaging. Indications for peripheral angiography include peripheral arterial disease (claudication, ischemia) or peripheral arterial trauma. Prior to the procedure, patients may be advised to hold antithrombotic medications (such as anticoagulants) for a few days. The procedure is similar to that for PCI and cardiac catheterization and is usually carried out under conscious sedation and local anesthetic. If obstruction is noted per angiography, balloon angioplasty may be carried out and one or more wire coils or stents placed to maintain patency of the arteries and improve blood flow. Following the procedure, pressure is applied to the insertion site to prevent bleeding and the patient is monitored carefully for complications to the procedure, which may include stroke, MI, hemorrhage, vascular trauma, and impaired circulation of extremity.

CARDIOVASCULAR SURGERY

Coronary artery bypass grafting (CABG) is typically performed on patients who have severe coronary artery disease in at least three vessels, or diffuse disease in the left main coronary artery.

Valve replacement is typically performed for severe valvular regurgitation or stenosis, or endocarditis. Surgery is typically considered for patients who do not respond to medical management efforts.

Cardiovascular surgery is indicated for congenital heart defects that may be present in either infants or adults.

Cardiac transplantation is performed on patients who have irreversible heart failure or cardiomyopathy. Because of the risks involved, cardiac transplantation is only performed after all other treatment options have been exhausted.

Surgical interventions, such Catheter Ablation, Cox Maze (Version IV), Wolf Mini-Maze, or Saltman Micromaze may be performed to treat cardiac dysrhythmias, such as atrial fibrillation with rapid ventricular response, Wolff-Parkinson-White Syndrome, and ventricular tachycardia that does not respond to medical management.

TEACHING

Prior to cardiac surgery, the patient should be given an overview of what will occur during the surgery, including the use of anesthesia, paralytics, mechanical ventilation, and use of the bypass machine. They should be informed about the importance of activity following the surgery, as it will help prevent pneumonia and other complications. The patient should also be informed of the importance of coughing, deep breathing, and utilizing the incentive spirometer. Teaching should be provided regarding the importance of effective pain management. Patients need to understand that they will experience some pain after the surgery, and that effective pain management will be necessary to decrease anxiety and facilitate post-surgical activity.

TESTING

Prior to cardiac surgery, a complete history and physical will be performed. An ECG and chest X-ray will be obtained. Routine lab work, such as a complete blood count, basic metabolic panel, coagulation studies, and a blood type and screen cross-match will be obtained. If the patient is on anticoagulation therapy, medication will be held and surgery will not be performed until coagulation levels have normalized. Pulmonary function testing and arterial blood gases will be drawn to assess lung fitness. Carotid Doppler will be performed bilaterally to assess carotid patency.

> **Review Video: Blood Gases**
> Visit mometrix.com/academy and enter code: 611909

CORONARY ARTERY BYPASS GRAFTING

Coronary artery bypass grafting (CABG) is a surgical procedure in which a coronary artery that has been occluded with atherosclerotic plaque is removed and replaced with a patent vessel that has been harvested from another part of the body. The patient is given general anesthetic and a paralytic, and then placed on a mechanical ventilator during the procedure. During an "on-pump" CABG, the patient's blood is circulated through a cardiopulmonary bypass machine (CBM) to supplant the functions of the heart and lungs while the repair is being performed. The heart is then stopped for the procedure. During an "off-pump" CABG, blood flow is only stopped in the area in which the grafting is being performed.

The graft is typically harvested from the internal mammary artery, the radial artery, or the saphenous vein. Once harvested, the graft is attached to the aorta, creating an alternate pathway for coronary circulation. After the graft is in place, blood flow to the heart is restored.

RISKS

Patients who have received a coronary artery bypass graft (CABG) are at risk for complications typical to all surgeries, such as hypovolemia, bleeding, infection at the incision site, sepsis, pneumonia, and deep vein thrombosis.

There are also complications related specifically to the receipt of a CABG. Postperfusion syndrome, or "pump head", is a neurocognitive impairment that occurs as a result of on-pump CABG. Stroke may also occur as a result of thrombotic occlusion or hypoperfusion to the brain. Acute renal failure may also occur as a result of renal artery occlusion, or hypoperfusion.

VALVES USED IN A VALVE REPLACEMENT

Most mechanical valves are made of a graphite base coated with a biocompatible ceramic-like material, though some are made with metal and/or plastics. Although mechanical valves last the longest of the replacement valves, the patient will require continuous anticoagulation therapy to prevent clots from forming on the valve.

A tissue valve is one harvested from animal tissue and chemically treated to allow it to be implanted within a human. Many tissue valves have a stent that supports the valve and allows for ease of implantation. Though the tissue valve will not last as long as a mechanical valve, the patient will not require continued anticoagulation therapy after the surgery.

A homographic valve is harvested from a human donor. These are typically implanted in children with congenital birth defects, as they will not require long-term anticoagulation. Because they come from human donors, homographic valves provide the best hemodynamic performance. However, they can only be used to replace aortic or pulmonic valves. Furthermore, supplies of homographic valves are limited.

RISKS

Valve replacement surgery carries risks beyond those typically involved in undergoing other surgical procedures. For example, the patient is at risk of damage to the valve placement sutures if the patient's blood pressure becomes elevated. Therefore, the patient's blood pressure should be closely monitored and maintained below 120 mmHg to prevent damage from occurring. The patient is at an increased risk of developing atrial fibrillation and cardiac dysrhythmias such as ventricular tachycardia and heart block. Therefore, the patient's cardiac rhythm should be closely monitored, as well. A temporary pacemaker may be required if the patient develops symptomatic heart block, and amiodarone or lidocaine may be prescribed to control ventricular tachycardia.

After the placement of a mechanical valve, the patient has an increased risk for bleeding. This is primarily because of necessary anticoagulation therapy to prevent thrombus formation. Thus, coagulation studies should be closely monitored to ensure that anticoagulation medication is at a therapeutic level. The patient's blood count should also be closely monitored, as any sudden drop in hemoglobin or hematocrit may indicate bleeding which should be reported and treated.

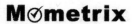

CARDIOVASCULAR SURGERY COMPLICATIONS

After cardiovascular surgery, the patient is at risk for a number of complications related to the cardiovascular and pulmonary systems. These complications can potentially be life threatening if they are not addressed quickly. Continuous cardiac monitoring and frequent evaluations of vital signs should be performed to rule out cardiac dysrhythmias, hypotension, hypertension, and ECG changes related to myocardial infarction. The patient's cardiac output should also be monitored, as a low cardiac output could be caused by bleeding or cardiac tamponade, and may lead to heart failure and acute renal failure. Pulmonary complications include pulmonary edema, pneumonia, and aspiration. The patient should also be monitored for other complications, such as stroke, ileus, and pancreatitis.

NURSING CONSIDERATIONS

There are a number of nursing activities that should be performed to ensure appropriate healing after cardiovascular surgery. Frequent cardiovascular and pulmonary assessments should be completed to ensure adequate perfusion and oxygenation. Any signs of complications such as cardiac dysrhythmias or respiratory complications should be reported and treated as soon as possible. The patient's pain should be adequately controlled to ensure otherwise difficult activities such as coughing, deep breathing, and ambulation take place. Ambulation should be undertaken as soon as possible, typically on the first postoperative day. Early ambulation helps to decrease the risk of deep vein thrombosis and pneumonia, and encourages the return of bowel function. Fluid balance should be closely monitored to prevent fluid overload.

DISCHARGE TEACHING

Prior to discharge, the patient should be given information regarding important lifestyle modifications to ensure good health. This includes the need for a heart-healthy diet and frequent exercise, decreased alcohol consumption, and smoking cessation. Incision care should be taught to prevent infection at the surgical site. Teaching regarding medications should be provided, including the reason for taking the medication, and proper medication times and dosages. The patient should be encouraged to follow up with their primary care physician for postoperative monitoring. If possible, the patient's family should be involved in postoperative teaching to facilitate their understanding of the discharge instructions. In this way, involved family members can also be supportive and assist the patient in maintaining treatment compliance. Written materials should be given to the patients to serve as reminders of what they were taught.

Cardiovascular Pharmacology

GLYCOPROTEIN IIB/IIIA INHIBITORS

Glycoprotein IIb/IIIa inhibitors function by blocking glycoprotein IIb/IIIa receptors. This prevents fibrinogen from binding and creating a thrombus. Glycoprotein IIb/IIIa inhibitors are indicated for patients diagnosed with acute coronary syndrome, or for those who are receiving a percutaneous coronary intervention (PCI).

Eptifibatide (Integrilin) is given as an IV bolus of 180 mcg/kg over 2 minutes. This is followed by a continuous IV infusion of 2 mcg/kg/min for up to 72 hours. Tirofiban (Aggrastat) is given as an IV bolus of 0.4 mcg/kg/min over 30 minutes, followed by a continuous IV infusion at 0.1 mcg/kg/min for 12 to 24 hours.

NURSING CONSIDERATIONS

Before infusing a glycoprotein IIb/IIIa inhibitor, a complete blood count, basic metabolic panel, and anticoagulation studies should be obtained to establish baseline levels. Intravenous access should be established peripherally in two places to ensure appropriate and timely access. Vital signs and neurological status should be checked prior to beginning therapy.

During therapy, the patient should be closely monitored for any signs or symptoms of bleeding. The patient's neurological status should be frequently assessed for any changes that might indicate intracerebral hemorrhage. The patient's cardiovascular status should be assessed for any signs of further ischemia, as this indicates that the antithrombotic therapy is ineffective.

DIURETICS

PHARMACOLOGIC EFFECT

Diuretics are a classification of medication that affects the nephron of the kidney, resulting in increased sodium and fluid excretion. Diuretics can affect the nephron in a variety of places, such as in the loop of Henle, the renal tubules, and the collecting ducts. Diuretics are indicated in patients who require close fluid management, such as in cases of heart failure, pulmonary edema, and idiopathic edema. It is also indicated in patients who require cardiac workload reductions, such as those with hypertension. Other conditions that may require diuretics include hepatic cirrhosis, hypercalcemia, nephrolithiasis, and nephrotic syndrome.

COMMONLY PRESCRIBED DIURETICS

Furosemide is a diuretic that can be given orally or intravenously. The most common oral dosage is 20 to 80mg; a maximum of 600 mg can be given daily. If the patient requires intravenous Furosemide, the typical dosage is between 10 and 40 mg given as an intravenous push either once or twice daily.

Hydrochlorothiazide is a diuretic that affects the distal renal tubule. It is only available as an oral medication. The minimum dosage is 25 mg per day, though a patient could safely receive as much as 200 mg per day.

Spironolactone is a potassium-sparing diuretic that affects the distal renal tubule and the collecting duct. The minimum dosage is 25 mg per day. Because of its long half-life, Spironolactone should only be prescribed once daily.

ADVERSE REACTIONS

The more common adverse reactions from diuresis result from excessive diuresis. When this occurs, the patient may become dehydrated and experience dizziness, nausea, vomiting, or orthostatic hypotension. They may also have signs or symptoms of hypernatremia, such as generalized weakness, muscle spasm, increased confusion, or lethargy.

Because many diuretics are non-potassium sparing, the patient may also develop hypokalemia, as a result of excessive potassium excretion. Further, the patient may show signs and symptoms of hypokalemia such as constipation, muscle cramping, decreased reflexes, and cardiac dysrhythmias.

Though rare, some patients may develop ototoxicity when receiving high doses of diuretics. Finally, there is also a risk that a patient may develop interstitial nephritis as a result of diuretic therapy.

CLASSES OF ANTIDYSRHYTHMIC DRUGS

Class	Actions	Indications
Class IA Sodium channel blockers (disopyramide, procainamide, quinidine)	Decrease myocardial excitability and conduction velocity and delay repolarization. Reduce/Eliminate ventricular ectopic foci stimulation. ECG: Widened QRS and prolonged QT.	AF, PACs, PVCs, VT, Wolff-Parkinson-White syndrome
Class IB Sodium channel blockers (Lidocaine, mexiletine, phenytoin)	Similar to IA but accelerate repolarization. Reduce/Eliminate ventricular ectopic foci stimulation. No significant effect on ECG.	PVCs, VT, VF, and digitalis-induced ventricular dysrhythmias.
Class IC Sodium channel blockers (Flecainide, propafenone)	Similar to IA and IB but stronger dysrhythmic action and depress cardiac conduction at Bundle of His/Purkinje. Reduce/Eliminate ventricular ectopic foci stimulation. ECG: Widened QRS and prolonged PR.	VT, SVT, AF, AFl, Wolff-Parkinson-White syndrome.
Class II Beta blockers (atenolol, esmolol, metoprolol, carvedilol, propranolol, acebutolol)	Myocardial depressants. Block beta-adrenergic stimulation, reduce activity of SA node, reduce/eliminate atrial ectopic foci stimulation. ECG: Prolonged PR and bradycardia.	SVT, VT, PVCs.
Class III Potassium channel blockers (amiodarone, dronedarone, dofetilide, ibutilide, sotalol	Delay repolarization. Prolong refractory period and myocardial action potential and block alpha and beta-adrenergic stimulation. ECG: Prolonged QT. Amiodarone and dronedarone prolong PR and widen QRS. Sotalol (which has class II properties) prolongs QT and PR and causes bradycardia. Dofetilide and ibutilide prolong QT.	Severe VT, VF and resistant AF and AFL.
Class IV Calcium channel blockers (verapamil, diltiazem	Prolong AV nodal effective refractory period, reduce AV nodal conduction, and rapid ventricular conduction associated with AF.	Paroxysmal SVT, AF and AFL rate control.

ELECTROLYTES FOR MANAGING SPECIFIC ARRHYTHMIAS

Electrolyte supplement	Arrhythmia and ECG changes related to low electrolyte levels
Potassium	Hypokalemia: Cardiac excitability with re-entrant arrhythmias, atrial tachycardia with block, VT, torsades de pointes, VF. ECG: P waves widen, PR interval prolong. QT interval may not be evident as t wave flattens or inverts, U waves develop. T and U waves may merge. ST segment depressed.
Calcium	Hypocalcemia: Specific arrhythmias are uncommon, but ECG changes may occur. ECG: ST segment and QT interval prolonged, T waves may flatten or invert but duration remains unchanged.
Magnesium	Hypomagnesemia: AV block and intraventricular conduction disturbances. No specific ECG changes are associated with hypomagnesia.

PHARMACOLOGIC EFFECTS FOR CALCIUM CHANNEL BLOCKERS

During cardiac muscle contraction, the calcium channels open a pathway to release a wave of calcium into the heart's myocyte cells to produce a contraction. Calcium channel blockers slow the rate of contraction by preventing the opening of these calcium channels. Because of their effectiveness in slowing myocyte contraction, calcium channel blockers such as Verapamil and Cardizem are typically prescribed to treat tachyarrhythmias.

Calcium channel blockers have a similar effect on arterial smooth muscle cells. This effect results in vasodilation and a decrease in cardiac afterload. For this reason, calcium channel blockers such as Norvasc and Plendil are also effective in treating hypertension and angina.

CONTRAINDICATIONS FOR PRESCRIBING CALCIUM CHANNEL BLOCKERS

Calcium channel blockers can have a synergistic effect when taken with beta-blockers. Therefore, they should be used carefully in patients who are already taking beta-blockers, as this synergistic effect might cause severe hypotension. Because calcium channel blockers slow conduction within the cardiac muscle cells, they should not be prescribed to patients with a history of atrioventricular block. They should also be used carefully in patients who have recently experienced a myocardial infarction, as studies have shown that they may increase mortality in this particular patient population

Calcium channel blockers are also effective vasodilators. Therefore, while taking them, some patients may complain of dizziness or headache, and may also experience peripheral edema.

ACE INHIBITORS

Angiotensin Converting Enzyme (ACE) inhibitors are prescribed to treat long-term heart conditions such as congestive heart failure, myocardial infarction, and hypertension. ACE inhibitors have also been found to improve long-term renal function in patients who have been diagnosed with diabetes.

However, ACE inhibitors are contraindicated in patients who are pregnant or breast-feeding. Further, if a patient develops angioedema while taking an ACE inhibitor (i.e., swelling beneath the skin, as opposed to a surface reaction such as welts), the medication should be discontinued immediately. Otherwise, the swelling may continue and occlude a patient's airway, as angioedema is predisposed to affect the head and neck, including the mouth, tongue, and larynx. ACE inhibitors should also be used cautiously in patients with aortic stenosis, hypertrophic cardiomyopathy, hypotension, hypovolemia, or renal or hepatic impairment.

INHIBITOR SIDE EFFECTS

The most common side effects involved in taking an Angiotensin Converting Enzyme (ACE) inhibitor include a dry cough, hypotension, and disturbances in the patient's sense of taste (i.e., gustatory changes). Other side effects may include dizziness, headache, fatigue, angina, tachycardia, and hyperkalemia. Male patients taking an ACE inhibitor may complain of impotence.

The patient should be instructed to take the appropriate dosage at the same time every day. They should be taught to exercise caution when sitting or standing, as hypotension may cause dizziness and increase the risk of falling. The patient should be instructed to notify their primary care physician if they experience symptoms of angioedema, including swelling around their lips, tongue or face, or if they have difficulty breathing.

ANGIOTENSIN II RECEPTOR BLOCKERS

Angiotensin II Receptor Blockers (ARBs) are prescribed in conjunction with Angiotensin Converting Enzyme (ACE) inhibitors to treat hypertension. They may also be prescribed to treat congestive heart failure in patients who are unable to tolerate ACE inhibitors.

ARBs are contraindicated in patients who are pregnant or breastfeeding. Extreme caution should be taken in patients who have a history of angioedema, as ARBs may cause an exacerbation of any angioedema symptoms. ARBs are also hepatotoxic and nephrotoxic. Therefore, they are contraindicated in patients who have been diagnosed with renal failure, cirrhosis of the liver, or liver failure.

SIDE EFFECTS

The most common side effects that may occur while in taking Angiotensin II Receptor Blockers (ARB) are dizziness, fatigue, and hypotension. ARBs may also cause headache, diarrhea, and hyperkalemia. Because ARBs can cause renal failure and hepatitis, patients should be closely monitored for any signs or symptoms or renal or liver impairment.

Patients should be instructed to take the appropriate dosage at the same time every day. They should be taught to be careful when sitting or standing, as hypotension may cause dizziness and increase their risk of falling. These patients should also be instructed on other lifestyle changes than can be made to lower their risk of complications related to hypertension.

PHARMACOLOGIC EFFECTS OF DIGOXIN

The pharmacologic effect of Digoxin is twofold. First, it increases the force of myocardial contractions. Second, it slows the heart rate by prolonging the refractory period of the AV node. Digoxin is indicated for patients in congestive heart failure, or those who have tachyarrhythmias, atrial fibrillation, and atrial flutter.

Digoxin is contraindicated in patients who have second- or third-degree atrioventricular block, or uncontrolled ventricular arrhythmias and as this may cause symptomatic bradycardia. It is also contraindicated in patients who have constrictive pericarditis or aortic stenosis. Care should be taken in patients with a history of electrolyte imbalances such as hypokalemia, hypercalcemia, and hypomagnesemia, as they are at increased risk for digoxin toxicity.

SIDE EFFECTS

The most common side effects experienced when taking digoxin include fatigue, bradycardia, anorexia, nausea, or vomiting. The patient may also complain of headache, blurred vision, or diarrhea. In addition, the patient may experience hyperkalemia, or thrombocytopenia. Further, while taking digoxin, the patient may experience ECG changes, sinoatrial block, or atrioventricular block or arrhythmias.

The patient should be instructed to take their digoxin as prescribed. They should understand that digoxin has a narrow therapeutic range (between 0.8 to 2 ng/mL), and will require frequent blood tests to ensure they are properly receiving a therapeutic amount of medication. The patient should be instructed of the signs and symptoms of digoxin toxicity.

TOXICITY

Digoxin toxicity occurs when the patient's digoxin level is above the therapeutic range. It is typically caused by dehydration, acute renal failure, or as the result of an electrolyte imbalance. There are a number of signs and symptoms related to digoxin toxicity. The patient may experience visual disturbances such as blurred vision, photophobia, or a yellow or green visual tint. They may experience nausea, vomiting, constipation, confusion, or severe abdominal pain. Patients with digoxin toxicity may also complain of itching or tingling in their extremities. ECG changes involved in digoxin toxicity include atrioventricular heart block, ventricular tachycardia, sinus bradycardia, or sinus arrest.

PHARMACOLOGIC EFFECTS OF DOPAMINE

Dopamine acts as a vasopressor and an inotropic agent (e.g., affecting the force of heart muscle contraction). It is given to increase blood pressure, and to increase cardiac output and urinary output. It is also prescribed in conjunction with fluid replacement therapy to treat shock.

The specific way in which it affects the patient is dependent upon the dosage. Low dose dopamine (0.5 to 3 mcg/kg/min) stimulates renal dopamine receptors, causing vasodilation within the kidney and increasing urine output (thus, sometimes referred to a "renal dose"). A medium dose of dopamine (3 to 10 mcg/kg/min) stimulates dopamine receptors and beta-adrenergic receptors, and reduces hypotension arising from poor cardiac output. High dose of dopamine (greater than 10mcg/kg/min) stimulates alpha-adrenergic receptors, and corrects hypotension due to poor systemic vascular resistance. How3ver, it also causes renal vasoconstriction and thus may injure the kidneys with prolonged use.

SIDE EFFECTS

Dopamine is contraindicated patients with tachyarrhythmias, as it has been known to elevate the patient's heart rate. It should be used cautiously in patients who are hypovolemic or who have recently had a myocardial infarction as it increases cardiac workload and oxygen demand. Dopamine should also be used cautiously in patients who are pregnant or breastfeeding.

The most common side effects are tachyarrhythmias, palpitations, and angina. The patient may also complain of a headache, dyspnea, nausea or vomiting. Close monitoring of a peripheral IV site is required, as dopamine is irritating to the vein.

PHARMACOLOGIC EFFECTS OF DOBUTAMINE

Dobutamine is a positive inotropic (heart contraction strengthening) agent that increases cardiac output by stimulating the myocardial beta-adrenergic receptors to increase contractility. Dobutamine can produce a mild increase in heart rate, blood pressure, and cardiac output. At the same time it will lower systemic vascular resistance and right atrial pressure. Dobutamine is typically prescribed for the short-term treatment of congestive heart failure. Intravenous infusions are routinely started at a low rate (0.5 to 1 mcg/kg/min) and titrated upward every few minutes until the desired effect is achieved. The usual range is 2 to 20 mcg/kg/min.

SIDE EFFECTS

Dobutamine is contraindicated in patients who have been diagnosed with aortic stenosis. It should be used cautiously in patients who have recently had a myocardial infarction, as it increases cardiac workload and oxygen consumption. It should also be used cautiously in patients who are in atrial fibrillation, as well as those who are hypovolemic, pregnant, or breastfeeding.

The most common side effects of dobutamine are hypertension, tachycardia, and premature ventricular contractions. The patient may also complain of palpitations, angina, or headache. Some patients may experience shortness of breath, nausea, or vomiting.

PHARMACOLOGIC EFFECTS OF MILRINONE

Milrinone is a phosphodiesterase inhibitor that increases contractility by increasing the availability of calcium within the cardiac muscle cell. It has a similar effect within the smooth muscles of the arteries, causing vasodilation. This results in decreased cardiac preload and afterload, and reduced systemic vascular resistance and right atrial pressure. Milrinone is typically prescribed to treat congestive heart failure in patients who did not respond to other vasodilators. Intravenous infusions are typically started at a 50 mcg/kg loading dose, followed by a continuous infusion at 0.5 mcg/kg/min. The typical range of milrinone is 0.375 to 0.75 mcg/kg/min.

SIDE EFFECTS

Milrinone is contraindicated in patients who have severe aortic or pulmonary valve disease. It should be used cautiously in patients who have a history of cardiac arrhythmias, electrolyte imbalances, or patients who are pregnant. A decreased dose may be required for patients with a history of renal impairment.

Patients who receive milrinone therapy are also at an increased risk of developing ventricular arrhythmias. The patient may complain of headache, nausea, vomiting and chest pain. Liver function tests should be closely monitored, as patients receiving milrinone may develop liver function abnormalities. The patient may also develop hypokalemia or thrombocytopenia.

PHARMACOLOGIC EFFECTS OF NOREPINEPHRINE

Norepinephrine has significant beta-adrenergic properties, causing increased cardiac muscle contractility and vasodilation of the coronary arteries. It also has strong alpha-adrenergic properties, causing vasoconstriction in the peripheral vasculature. Norepinephrine administration results in moderate increases in heart rate, mean arterial blood pressure, systemic vascular resistance, and right atrial pressure, coupled with a decrease in cardiac output. Norepinephrine is indicated for the treatment of hypotension secondary to myocardial infarction, septic shock, and certain drug reactions. The typical range for administering norepinephrine is between 1 and 40 mcg/min, titrated upward every few minutes until the desires effect is achieved.

SIDE EFFECTS

Prolonged hypertension resulting from norepinephrine administration should be avoided, as it may cause tissue ischemia and organ failure. Ideally, norepinephrine should be infused through a central line. If norepinephrine is being infused peripherally, the site should be carefully monitored as it may cause damage to the vein. Extravasation (medication escaping from the infusion vessel) may cause necrosis of the tissue surrounding the site and subsequent "purple glove syndrome" (severe swelling of an extremity (such as a hand) to the point of discoloration and pain – which may lead to amputation). If extravasation does take place, phentolamine should be given subcutaneously around the site to prevent the development of necrosis.

Patients who receive norepinephrine may complain of headache or increased anxiety. They may also experience shortness of breath and bradycardia.

PHARMACOLOGIC EFFECTS OF VASOPRESSIN

Vasopressin increases cardiac preload by altering the permeability of the renal collecting ducts to increase water reabsorption, thereby increasing systemic vascular volume. It also increases peripheral vasoconstriction by stimulating V1 receptors in the vascular smooth muscles. This results in moderate increases in blood pressure, systemic vascular resistance, and right atrial pressure. Vasopressin is indicated for the treatment of diabetes insipidus, and to manage hypotension secondary to septic shock. Further, a one-time dose of vasopressin can be given as part of ACLS guidelines for the treatment of pulseless ventricular tachycardia or ventricular fibrillation.

The typical dosage of vasopressin is 5 to 10 units given 2 to 3 times daily. The dosage of vasopressin that is given to treat pulseless VF/VT is 40 units as an IV push.

SIDE EFFECTS

Vasopressin is contraindicated in patients who have a history of chronic renal failure. It should be used cautiously in patients who have a history of seizures, asthma, heart failure, and renal impairment.

Patients who are receiving vasopressin may complain of dizziness, chest pain, abdominal pain, nausea, and vomiting. They may experience paleness, diaphoresis, or fever. Patients receiving higher doses of vasopressin are at an increased risk of developing water intoxication or congestive heart failure. Therefore, the patient's fluid status should be carefully monitored while receiving vasopressin and any significant fluid overload should be addressed.

PHARMACOLOGIC EFFECTS OF NITROPRUSSIDE

Nitroprusside is a vasodilator that works by relaxing smooth muscle tone in the arterial and venous vasculature. Nipride may result in a mild increase in heart rate, and a moderate decrease in blood pressure, systemic vascular resistance and right atrial pressure. Nitroprusside is indicated for the treatment of hypertensive crisis. It is also effective in treating cardiogenic shock because of its effectiveness in lowering cardiac preload and afterload. A nitroprusside drip is started at a rate of 0.3 mcg/kg/min. It can be titrated to achieve the desired affect up to a maximum dosage of 10 mcg/kg/min.

CYANIDE TOXICITY

Cyanide can be released from nitroprusside when incubated with a variety of biological materials, including blood. Thus, cyanide toxicity can occur after prolonged exposure to high doses of nitroprusside. This results in decreased cellular respiration, and causes a shift in cells from aerobic to anaerobic metabolic processes. The presence of cyanide toxicity can be measured by checking lactic acid levels.

Common signs and symptoms involved in cyanide toxicity include generalized weakness, seizures, shortness of breath, confusion, and coma. The patient may complain of nausea, vomiting, headache, and abdominal pain. If the patient starts to show any signs or symptoms of cyanide toxicity, nitroprusside should be weaned and discontinued, or replaced with a different vasodilator agent.

SIDE EFFECTS

Nitroprusside is contraindicated in patients who have diminished cerebral perfusion, as a low blood pressure may lead to further cerebral tissue damage. Nitroprusside should be used cautiously in patients with renal or hepatic impairment as cyanide toxicity may cause further liver or kidney damage. It should also be used cautiously in patients who are hyponatremic or who have been diagnosed with hypothyroidism.

The most common side effects experienced when taking nitroprusside are dizziness, headache, abdominal pain, and nausea. Patients may also complain of palpitations, blurred vision, restlessness, or dyspnea. A nitroprusside drip should not be allowed to infuse for more than 48 hours, as it increases the patient's risk for cyanide toxicity.

PHARMACOLOGIC EFFECTS OF INTRAVENOUS NITROGLYCERINE

Nitroglycerine works by stimulating the release of nitric oxide from the endothelial lining of the veins, resulting in vasodilation. This can result in a mild increase in heart rate, as well as a moderate decrease in blood pressure, stroke volume, systemic vascular resistance, and right atrial pressure. It is the medication of choice used in the treatment of cardiac ischemia, pulmonary edema, and congestive heart failure.

A nitroglycerine drip is typically started at a rate of 10 mcg/min. It can be titrated upward by 10 mcg/min every 10 minutes until the desired effect is achieved.

SIDE EFFECTS

Because nitroglycerin increases venous capacitance and reduces stroke volume, it is contraindicated in patients whose cardiac output is impaired, such as in cases of constrictive pericarditis or pericardial tamponade. It should be used cautiously in patients with cerebral hemorrhage as it may significantly decrease cerebral perfusion. It should also be used cautiously in cases of severe liver impairment, hypovolemia, and hypertrophic cardiomyopathy.

The most common side effects are dizziness, hypotension, and tachycardia. Some patients may also complain of severe headaches, which may occur secondary to venous pressure on involved nerves. The patient may also experience restlessness, blurred vision, syncope, flushing, nausea, and vomiting.

PHARMACOLOGIC EFFECTS OF NICARDIPINE

Nicardipine is a medication that causes vasodilation by inhibiting calcium absorption within the myocardial and vascular smooth muscle cells. This interrupts the usual excitation-contraction cycle and prevents vasoconstriction. Nicardipine is indicated for hypertensive crises, Prinzmetal's angina (aka, angina inversa), and the management of congestive heart failure. It is the medication of choice for controlling hypertension in a patient with neurological injuries.

A nicardipine drip is typically started at 5 mg/hr, and titrated upward every 15 minutes until the desired blood pressure is achieved. The maximum dosage is 15 mg/hr. The half-life is 2 to 4 hours.

SIDE EFFECTS

Nicardipine is contraindicated in patients with a history of sick sinus syndrome or atrioventricular block, as it may cause longer conduction delays. It is also contraindicated in patients with a systolic blood pressure less than 90 mmHg, as it will cause severe hypotension. Nicardipine should be used cautiously in patients with severe renal or hepatic impairment, as decreased perfusion secondary to hypotension may cause worsening organ failure.

The most common side effect of nicardipine is peripheral edema. The patient should also be monitored for any cardiac dysrhythmias or congestive heart failure. Some patients may complain of headache, blurred vision, dyspnea, or dry mouth.

Electrophysiologic Interventions

PACEMAKERS
HEART RHYTHM SOCIETY'S PACEMAKER CODES

The Heart Rhythm Society (HRS) –known prior to 2004 as the North American Society of Pacing and Electrophysiology (NASPE) – issues standardized codes which are used to indicate and describe a patient's pacemaker settings. The first coded letter indicates which chamber of the heart is paced. O means none, A means atrium, V means ventricle, and D means both the atrium and the ventricle. The second letter indicates which chamber is sensed, and the same codes O, A, V and D apply. The third letter indicates how the pacemaker will respond to sensing. O means none, T means a stimulus is triggered, I means the heart beat was adequate so the stimulus was inhibited, and D means a stimulus may or may not have been inhibited, depending upon the situation. The fourth letter indicates other available programming features. O means none, P means it is programmable with either one or two parameters, M means it is programmable with more than two parameters, C means it is being interrogated, and R is rate modulation depending on certain parameters.

PACEMAKER FUNCTION

Pacemaker function is dependent upon its ability to sense the patient's intrinsic heart rhythm, and its subsequent ability to capture a heartbeat. While sensing the patient's heart rhythm, the pacemaker measures the electrical activity in the heart. The range of millivolts that the pacemaker can sense (its sensitivity) is programmed into the device during implantation. If the electroconductivity of the heart falls below the range of sensitivity, the pacemaker will respond, initiating an electrical stimulus to trigger systole. The pacemaker settings can be easily changed, as needed, to support appropriate perfusion.

SINGLE AND DUAL CHAMBER PACEMAKERS AND BI-VENTRICULAR SYSTEMS

A single chamber pacemaker has one lead to stimulate either an atrium or a ventricle. A dual chamber pacemaker has two leads, to stimulate an atrium and a ventricle. Patients with severe congestive heart failure may require a bi-ventricular pacing system. It is indicated for patients who have a lack of coordination in ventricular contraction, leading to decreased ventricular filling time and reduced stroke volume. During bi-ventricular pacing, ventricular contraction is stimulated using leads placed in the right ventricle and coronary sinus. Bi-ventricular systems are indicated for patients who have an ejection fraction less than 35%, and are already receiving optimal levels of congestive heart failure (CHF) medication.

PERMANENT PACEMAKER

A permanent pacemaker is a device that is implanted in the patient to increase the patient's heart rate if their natural rhythm is too slow to provide adequate perfusion. It is typically placed in patients who have symptomatic bradycardia that is refractory to medical management. Symptomatic bradycardia typically results from a sinus node abnormality or from an atrioventricular block.

A permanent pacemaker may also be indicated for patients whose heart is unable to compensate for increased demand. States of severe left ventricular dysfunction, including cases of severe congestive heart failure, may also require placement of a pacemaker.

TRANSVENOUS PACEMAKERS

Transvenous pacemakers, comprised of a catheter with a lead at the end, are a temporary pacemaker that may be used prophylactically or therapeutically on a temporary basis to treat a cardiac abnormality, especially bradycardia. The catheter is inserted through a vein at the femoral or neck area and attached to an external pulse generator. Clinical uses include:

- To treat persistent dysrhythmias not responsive to medications.
- To increase cardiac output with bradydysrhythmia by increasing rate.
- To decrease ventricular or supraventricular tachycardia by "overdrive" stimulation of contractions.
- To treat secondary heart block caused by myocardial infarction, ischemia, and drug toxicity.
- To improve cardiac output after cardiac surgery.
- To provide diagnostic information through electrophysiology studies, which induce dysrhythmias for purposes of evaluation.
- To provide pacing when a permanent pacemaker malfunctions.

Complications are similar to implanted pacemakers and include increased risk of pacemaker syndrome.

TRANSCUTANEOUS PACING

Transcutaneous pacing is used temporarily to treat bradydysrhythmia that doesn't respond to medications (atropine) and results in hemodynamic instability. Generally, an arterial line is placed and the patient provided oxygen before the pacing. The placement of pacing pads (large self-adhesive pads) and ECG leads varies somewhat according to the type of equipment, but usually one pacing pad (negative) is placed on the left chest, inferior to the clavicle, and the other (positive) on the left back, inferior to the scapula, so the heart is sandwiched between the two pads so that the myocardium is depolarized through the chest wall. Lead wires attach the pads to the monitor. The rate of pacing is usually set between 60 and 70 bpm. Current is increased slowly until capture occurs—a spiking followed by QRS sequence—then the current is readjusted downward if possible just to maintain capture. Both demand and fixed modes are available, but demand mode is preferred. Patients may require analgesia, especially if a higher current setting is needed.

PACEMAKER PLACEMENT COMPLICATIONS

Possible complications following pacemaker placement include bleeding, infection, cardiac tamponade, or a collapsed lung. Rare pacemaker-specific complications include generator failure (very rare) and lead failure (less rare). To ensure proper function, the patient should be placed on cardiac telemetry to monitor for arrhythmias. Care should be taken to make sure that ECG leads are not placed on top of the pacemaker. The surgical site should be carefully monitored for bleeding or the development of a hematoma. The patient should be frequently assessed for any signs or symptoms of cardiac tamponade, which may occur from perforation of the pericardium during lead placement. The patient should also be monitored for any thromboembolic syndromes such as pulmonary embolism or stroke. The patient should be monitored for any signs of infection, as it may lead to pericarditis. Prophylactic antibiotics may be prescribed to prevent infection.

CARING FOR A PATIENT AFTER PACEMAKER IMPLANTATION

The patient should be kept on bed rest for 6 to 12 hours postoperatively, depending upon the patient's condition and relevant institutional policy. Arm movement on the side in which the pacemaker has been implanted should be limited to prevent migration of the pacing wires. The patient may have their arm placed in a sling to aid in limiting movement. The insertion site should be carefully monitored for bleeding or hematoma. Prior to discharge, the patient should have a chest radiograph to confirm proper lead placement.

Discharge teaching should include information regarding any activity restrictions in the affected arm. The patient should be given information about the type of pacemaker they have received and its proper pacing settings.

CARDIAC ABLATION PROCEDURE

Cardiac ablation procedure includes:

- Pretesting: Blood tests (may vary) and ECG is carried out.
- All usual heart and blood pressure medication are usually taken in the morning before the procedure unless otherwise advised by physician.
- Patient should ingest only water the morning of the test and no fluids for 3 to 6 hours before test.
- IV line is placed in the arm for administration of anesthetic agent and fluids and ECG monitoring electrodes applied.

- Patient is transported to the electrophysiology laboratory, placed on the table, and draped. For A-fib, defibrillation pads are applied to the patient's back.
- Conscious sedation is administered. Heavier sedation is usually needed for A-fib ablation.
- Local anesthetic is applied to catheter insertion sites (commonly femoral artery or vein). For long procedures, a urinary catheter is inserted.
- Three catheters (intracardiac ultrasound for viewing, ablation catheter, and mapping catheter to detect electrical activity) are inserted and advanced into the heart. For A-fib ablation, 5 catheters are inserted, 3 in one femoral vein or artery and 2 in the other.
- Ablation procedures are carried out, using heat (radiofrequency) and/or cold (cryotherapy) to scar the tissue, interfering with transmission of impulses.
- Catheters are removed, compression applied to prevent bleeding, and patient monitored for complications.

INDICATIONS AND POST-OPERATIVE CARE

Cardiac ablation is a minimally invasive procedure to treat atrial fibrillation and SVT uncontrolled by medications. Cardiac ablation is used for cardiac rhythm disorders (supraventricular tachycardia/arrhythmias) arising from the atria, including AV nodal reentry tachycardia (AVNRT), atrioventricular reentrant tachycardia (AVRT), atrial tachycardia (AT), and atrial flutter (AFL) as well as atrial fibrillation (A-fib). A-fib ablation (pulmonary vein isolation procedure) is more complex because the catheters must be positioned in the left atrium, and the procedure may need to be repeated more than once. Serious complications (such as hemorrhage, stroke, or MI) are rare. Following the procedure, the patient is monitored in the recovery room. Once stable, the patient is returned to the room. The patient must remain in supine position with head elevated no more than 30 degrees for 4 to 6 hours and must be advised to avoid crossing the legs. A compression dressing or device is placed at the insertion site(s) to prevent bleeding, and the sites must be assessed frequently.

CARDIOVERSION

Cardioversion is a timed electrical stimulation to the heart to convert a tachydysrhythmia (such as atrial fibrillation) to a normal sinus rhythm. Usually anticoagulation therapy is done for at least 3 weeks prior to elective cardioversion to reduce the risk of emboli, and digoxin is discontinued for at least 48 hours prior to cardioversion. During the procedure, the patient is usually sedated and/or anesthetized. Electrodes in the form of gel-covered paddles or pads are positioned on the left chest and left back (in front of and behind the heart), connected by leads to a computerized ECG and cardiac monitor with a defibrillator. The defibrillator is synchronized with the ECG so that the electrical current is delivered during ventricular depolarization (QRS). The timing must be precise in order to prevent ventricular tachycardia or ventricular fibrillation. Sometimes, drug therapy is used in conjunction with cardioversion; for example, antiarrhythmics (Cardizem®, Cordarone®) may be given before the procedure to slow the heart rate.

EMERGENCY DEFIBRILLATION

Emergency defibrillation is done to treat acute ventricular fibrillation or ventricular tachycardia in which there is no audible or palpable pulse. A higher voltage is generally used for defibrillation than is used for cardioversion, causing depolarization of myocardial cells, which can then repolarize to regain a normal sinus rhythm. Defibrillation delivers an electrical discharge usually through paddles applied to both sides of the chest. Defibrillation may be repeated, usually up to 3 times, at increasing voltage, but if the heart has not regained a sinus rhythm by then, cardiopulmonary resuscitation and advanced life support is required. Medications, such as epinephrine or vasopressin may be administered and cardiopulmonary resuscitation continued for one minute, after which defibrillation is again attempted. Additional medications, such as Cordarone®, magnesium, or procainamide, may be necessary if there are persistent ventricular dysrhythmias.

IMPLANTABLE CARDIOVERTER-DEFIBRILLATOR
FUNCTIONS

An implantable cardioverter-defibrillator (ICD) is a device that is capable of sensing and treating tachyarrhythmias. It consists of a series of leads positioned within the heart and attached to a battery system. When the device is implanted, it is programmed with a rate threshold number. If the patient's heart rate exceeds the rate threshold, the ICD will elicit a shock to return the heart rhythm to a slower rhythm. In this way an ICD has the ability to cardiovert a patient in atrial fibrillation with rapid ventricular response, and to defibrillate a patient in ventricular tachycardia or ventricular fibrillation. It can also provide pacing for episodes of bradyarrhythmia.

INDICATIONS

The primary indication for the placement of an implantable cardioverter-defibrillator (ICD) is cardiac arrest from ventricular fibrillation, or ventricular tachycardia that is refractory to medication management. The patient may be a candidate for ICD placement if they have a positive electrophysiology study combined with syncope. The patient may also require an ICD to prevent life threatening arrhythmias if they have had a significant myocardial infarction resulting in a low ejection fraction. Other conditions that may indicate the placement of an ICD include hypertrophic cardiomyopathy, right ventricular dysplasia, and Brugada syndrome.

TEACHING AFTER AN ICD PLACEMENT

The patient should be taught to limit activity in the arm on the side where the implantable cardioverter-defibrillator (ICD) was placed for a few weeks after surgery. The patient should also monitor the surgery site for any signs or symptoms of infection, and should notify their doctor if an infection occurs. The patient is typically instructed not to drive for 3 to 6 months after placement of an ICD, in order to ensure effectiveness in treating cardiac arrest related to ventricular tachycardia or ventricular fibrillation. The patient's ability to work is dependent upon their occupation and the level of activity they are required to perform their job. If the patient requires an order to perform light duty, it should be addressed with the doctor prior to discharge. The patient should also carry an identification card that provides information about the ICD.

ELECTRICAL DISCHARGES OF AN ICD

If the patient develops a life-threatening cardiac dysrhythmia, they may feel dizziness, lightheadedness, or palpitations secondary to the dysrhythmia. The resulting shock elicited by the implantable cardioverter-defibrillator (ICD) may or may not be felt. If the shock is felt, however, the patient may describe it as a jolting sensation – sometimes severe enough to warrant the description "being kicked in the chest." If the patient feels the ICD discharge multiple times, or if they continue to feel syncope or chest pain, they should go to the hospital immediately.

The patient's family members should be taught to initiate CPR if the patient is found unresponsive. They should also be informed that it is safe to touch the patient while the ICD is firing, as the shocks are mild enough externally that they will not cause the family member harm.

The patient should be instructed to have their ICD "interrogated" (checked for responsiveness) every 3 months to ensure it is working properly.

WEARABLE CARDIOVERTER DEFIBRILLATOR

A **wearable cardioverter defibrillator** (such as a LifeVest®) is a non-invasive defibrillator that operates automatically and does not require the assistance of a second person. The LifeVest® is used to prevent sudden cardiac death (SCD) in patients who are increased risk. It may be used temporarily while awaiting implantation of an ICD or for prolonged periods if not a candidate. Indications include heart failure with EF <35%, survival of previous cardiac arrest related to VT/VF, and arrhythmias post MI. Patients who are in the 3-month waiting period while attempting other therapy, <40 days post MI, awaiting heart transplantation, or have life expectancy of <1 year are candidates for the wearable cardioverter defibrillator. The vest has electrodes to monitor heart function and treatment pads to deliver shocks. The vest is placed next to the skin and secured snugly. A gong alarm alerts the patient that some problem is occurring, such as too loose vest. If the device detects a shockable rhythm, the vibration alert occurs, followed by siren alert, and voice prompts. The patient can press the response buttons to stop the shock. The shocking electrodes automatically release conductive gel and a treatment shock occurs.

Pulmonary Patient Care

Acute Pulmonary Embolus

PATHOPHYSIOLOGY

In cases of **pulmonary embolism (PE),** circulation in the pulmonary artery becomes blocked, most typically by a thrombus (although the embolus could also be tissue fragments, clumps of bacteria, protozoan parasites, fatty tissue released by a broken long bone, gas bubbles, etc.). Cancer may also cause a pulmonary embolism when a piece of cancerous tissue is dislodged from a tumor. A thrombus-generated embolus usually forms in the legs through deep vein thrombosis (DVT) or in the heart during atrial fibrillation or by way of a valvular disorder.

Once it is in the lungs, the thrombus occludes a branch of the pulmonary artery, decreasing the circulation of oxygenated blood. This can lead to severe hypoxemia and heart failure. If it is not treated quickly, a large PE can be fatal.

SIGNS AND SYMPTOMS

The classic signs and symptoms of a pulmonary embolism (PE) are pleuritic chest pain, dyspnea, and hemoptysis. A delay may occur in treating PE because these symptoms are shared with a number of other acute conditions, and because all three of the symptoms rarely occur at the same time. If other possible causes have been ruled out, then PE should be suspected. The patient may also experience jugular venous distension, a pleural rub, tachycardia, hypotension, and cyanosis in the lips and fingertips. Further, the patient may experience increased agitation, shortness of breath, and low oxygen saturation.

DIAGNOSIS

Pulmonary embolism (PE) is most often diagnosed using a computed tomography (CT) scan or an MRI. Both are noninvasive tests that utilize intravenous contrast dye to directly visualize the arterial circulation within the lung. With both a CT scan and an MRI, the clot can be quickly located.

Other tests can be done to rule out other conditions with similar symptoms. An ECG can be done to rule out acute MI. An arterial blood gas can be done to assess the patient's oxygenation status and rule out respiratory failure. A chest X-ray will rule out pneumothorax or hemothorax.

NURSING INTERVENTIONS

One of the primary nursing goals is prevention of pulmonary embolism (PE). Because many cases of PE occur as a result of a deep vein thrombosis (DVT), preventing a DVT will prevent the occurrence of a PE. The patient should be encouraged to walk frequently, or to perform leg exercises in the bed if they are unable to ambulate. A sequential compression device (SCD) may be applied to the legs to prevent the formation of a DVT. The patient should be frequently assessed for signs of a DVT, such as edema, redness or warmth in the lower extremities. If these are noted, the patient should be started on anticoagulation therapy.

In the case of recurrent PE, the patient may require the placement of an inferior vena cava (IVC) filter, which prevents any clots that form in the legs from reaching the lungs.

TREATMENTS

The primary goal of treatment in cases of pulmonary embolism (PE) is to reestablish circulation within the pulmonary vascular system. The patient may be started on intravenous thrombolytic therapy to break down the clot. If the clot is causing significant distress, an emergent embolectomy may be done to surgically to remove the clot. Once the clot has been removed, the patient will be started on anticoagulants to prevent a future PE from occurring.

While the patient is being treated for PE, they should also be placed on bed rest to prevent further stress on the heart. Adequate oxygen must be provided, and, if necessary, the patient may be sedated and intubated.

Acute Respiratory Distress Syndrome

Acute respiratory distress syndrome (ARDS) is a serious condition that develops in response to lung injury. It is characterized by a sudden buildup of fluid within the lungs, combined with an increase in alveolar permeability. This causes the alveoli and pulmonary capillaries to either collapse or fill with fluid. The result is a marked decline in oxygenation, resulting in respiratory distress. At the same time, there is a systemic inflammatory response that can lead to hypoxemia and multi-organ failure. If it is not treated quickly and appropriately, ARDS can be fatal.

RISK FACTORS

Acute respiratory distress syndrome (ARDS) is typically caused by either a direct injury to the lungs or by a severe insult to the body. Aspiration of gastric secretions is the most common cause of ARDS. The patient may also develop ARDS as a result of a bacteria or viral pneumonia, or through a blood-borne sepsis. ARDS may also develop from exposure to radiation or from chest trauma. Patients who have received multiple blood transfusions should be closely monitored for ARDS, as well. Patients who inhaled caustic chemicals such as ammonia or chlorine are also at risk.

SIGNS AND SYMPTOMS

Patients who develop acute respiratory distress syndrome (ARDS) typically experience a sudden onset of associated symptoms. These include shortness of breath, cyanosis, and tachypnea. The patient may also experience a persistent cough, and a low-grade fever. The patient will have a low oxygen saturation that does not respond to supplemental oxygen – even 100% oxygen – as a result of poor perfusion in the alveoli and capillaries. On a chest X-ray film, the patient's lungs will typically appear to be completely "white," as the accumulation of fluid impedes the passage of the Roentgen rays (x-rays). In the absence of complete "white out", multiple pleural effusions will be visualized.

TREATMENT

Patients who are diagnosed with acute respiratory distress syndrome (ARDS) are typically placed on a ventilator with additional positive end-expiratory pressure (PEEP) to prevent further alveolar collapse. While the patient is on the ventilator, intravenous sedation is provided to encourage comfort and decrease oxygen demand. While the patient is intubated, steps must be taken to prevent the onset of ventilator-associated pneumonia, which can increase the mortality rate of ARDS by up to 85%.

The patient's fluid balance must also be carefully maintained. Too little fluid will cause a decrease in preload and cardiac output, while too much fluid will cause additional fluid buildup within the lungs. Thus, it is not uncommon to provide both fluid boluses and diuretics over a short period of time in order to maintain a normovolemic state.

NURSING IMPLICATIONS

There are a number of nursing implications involved in the care of a patient with acute respiratory distress syndrome (ARDS). It is important to ensure that steps are taken to prevent ventilator-associated pneumonia (VAP), which can increase risk of mortality by as much as 85%. Keeping the head of the patient's bed higher than 30 degrees, and appropriate suctioning and mouth care can help prevent VAP. It is also important to combine additional nursing activities to decrease oxygen demand.

Fluid intake and output must be carefully maintained, to ensure appropriate fluid balance. If the patient becomes either fluid overloaded or hypovolemic, steps must be taken to restore the patient to a euvolemic state.

Acute Respiratory Failure

Respiratory failure refers to the inability of the respiratory system to maintain appropriate gas exchange. Chronic respiratory failure develops over a period of several days, while acute respiratory failure (ARF) can occur over the course of minutes to hours.

ARF is further divided into two categories: hypoxemic respiratory failure and hypercapnic respiratory failure. In hypoxemic respiratory failure, the lungs are unable to supply an adequate amount of oxygen to the blood. Patients with hypoxemic respiratory failure have a PaO_2 level less than 60 mm Hg. In hypercapnic respiratory failure, the lungs are unable to remove an appropriate amount of carbon dioxide from the blood stream. Patients experiencing hypercapnic respiratory failure have a PCO_2 level greater than 50 mm Hg.

CAUSES OF HYPERCAPNIC ACUTE RESPIRATORY FAILURE

Hypercapnic respiratory failure results in the inability of the respiratory system to remove an appropriate amount of carbon dioxide (CO2). Hypercapnic respiratory failure can result from conditions that cause a decreased respiratory rate, such as drug overdose, metabolic alkalosis, CNS infections, or hypothyroidism.

Hypercapnic respiratory failure can also be caused by an increased resistance to breathing, such as in cases of COPD exacerbation, asthma, muscle fatigue, or left ventricular failure.

Conditions which decrease the amount of area available for gas exchange can also lead to a hypercapnic and hypoxemic state, such as in abdominal disorders that affect diaphragm movement, or emphysema

CAUSES OF HYPOXEMIC RESPIRATORY FAILURE

During hypoxemic respiratory failure, the amount of oxygen perfusing the alveolar membrane is not enough to meet the body's needs.

The most common cause of hypoxemic respiratory failure is pneumonia or ARDS. Both conditions cause the alveoli become partially or completely collapsed or filled with fluid. This reduces the amount of oxygen that crosses the alveolar membrane to enter the blood stream.

Airway obstruction such as asthma, COPD, or choking, can also cause hypoxemic respiratory failure. This results in a decrease in the amount of oxygen available for perfusion.

Other conditions that can cause hypoxemic respiratory failure include pulmonary fibrosis, pulmonary embolism, and pneumothorax.

DIAGNOSIS

Acute respiratory failure (ARF) is diagnosed primarily using arterial blood gas (ABG) testing. Using an ABG sample, the patient's PO_2, PCO_2, pH, and sodium bicarbonate levels can be measured. This can also provide clues as to what is causing the respiratory failure.

A complete blood count can be done to assess the patient's hemoglobin. An elevated white blood cell count will indicate infection, such as pneumonia.

Other tests can be used to identify the cause of ARF. These include a lumbar puncture to check for CNS infection, a CT scan or chest X-ray to assess lung structure and the presence of any fluid, and toxicology screens to monitor for any drugs that might cause respiratory depression.

SIGNS AND SYMPTOMS

The most common symptoms of acute respiratory failure (ARF) are dyspnea and shortness of breath.

In cases of hypoxemic respiratory failure, the patient may experience increased confusion, tachycardia, hypertension, cyanosis, and cardiac dysrhythmias. The patient will also show signs of being unable to breathe, such as using their accessory muscles during inspiration, or having flared nostrils.

Patients with hypercapnic respiratory failure may complain of a headache or blurred vision. They may feel drowsy, or be difficult to arouse. The patient may also have asterixis (a flapping-like tremor that can be visualized when the patient extends their hands at the wrists).

CARING FOR A PATIENT WITH ACUTE RESPIRATORY FAILURE

The patient's wishes regarding mechanical ventilation should be clarified as promptly as possible (many patients have advanced directives foregoing it). The patient's pulse oximetry, heart rate, and blood pressure should be carefully monitored. Electrolyte analyses and a complete blood count should be repeated regularly, and any abnormal results should be reported. The patient's mental status should be assessed regularly, as a sudden decrease in mentation could indicate declining oxygenation. Similarly, the patient should be monitored for increased anxiety secondary to decreased oxygenation, as this can lead to agitation and a worsening hypoxemic state.

If the patient is intubated, nursing activities should be grouped together to decrease additional oxygen demand. Frequent mouth care and suctioning should be done to prevent ventilator-associated pneumonia.

TREATMENT

The primary goals in treating acute respiratory failure (ARF) are to restore appropriate gas exchange while treating the underlying cause and preventing further complications.

The patient may require supplemental oxygen. In cases of severe hypoxemia, the patient may need to be sedated and intubated. The patient should be placed on bed rest to reduce unnecessary oxygen demands. If the respiratory failure was caused by an infection, antibiotic therapy should be considered. If the respiratory failure was caused by an electrolyte imbalance, the patient's electrolytes should be closely monitored and replaced.

The patient may be given nitrates to control chest pain secondary to respiratory distress, and diuretics to decrease cardiac preload burdens. The patient may also be prescribed intravenous morphine to control pain and anxiety.

Other Pulmonary Disorders

PNEUMOTHORAX

During line placement, there is a risk that the insertion needle will pierce the lung, causing it to collapse. The patient is particularly at risk for developing a pneumothorax during a line placement in the subclavian or jugular vein.

Signs and symptoms of pneumothorax include sudden onset shortness of breath, cyanosis, pleural chest pain, and a dry cough. The patient may also experience a sudden drop in oxygen saturation. If the patient remains in a state of low oxygen saturation for an extended period of time, their level of consciousness may become decreased. Lung expansion will usually appear to be asymmetrical during inspiration, as well. Lung sounds may also be diminished or absent on the side in which the pneumothorax has occurred.

> **Review Video: Pneumothorax**
> Visit mometrix.com/academy and enter code: 186841
>
> **Review Video: Different Types of Lung Sounds**
> Visit mometrix.com/academy and enter code: 765616

DIAGNOSIS AND TREATMENT

If the lung sounds on the affected side are diminished or absent, a pneumothorax should be suspected. An arterial blood gas (ABG) can be done to assess the patient's oxygenation status. A chest X-ray can be done to visualize the presence of air outside of the lung.

Treatment may not be required if the pneumothorax is small, as it may resolve itself over time. However, if the pneumothorax is too large to resolve independently, a chest tube may be placed to remove the accumulated air from around the lung in the pleural cavity. This will restore an appropriate level expansion capacity for the lung. While the pneumothorax is present, the patient may require adjunctive oxygen.

HEMOTHORAX

Hemothorax occurs with bleeding into the pleural space, usually from major vascular injury such as tears in intercostal vessels, lacerations of great vessels, or trauma to lung parenchyma. A small bleed may be self-limiting and seal, but a tear in a large vessel can result in massive bleeding, followed quickly by hypovolemic shock. The pressure from the blood may result in inability of the lung to ventilate and a mediastinal shift. Often a hemothorax occurs with a pneumothorax, especially in severe chest trauma. Further symptoms include severe respiratory distress, decreased breath sounds, and dullness on auscultation. Diagnosis is per upright chest X-ray and sometimes CT and/or ultrasound. Treatment includes placement of a chest tube to drain the hemothorax, but with large volumes, the pressure may be preventing exsanguination, which can occur abruptly as the blood drains and pressure is reduced, so a large bore intravenous line should be in place and typed and cross-matched blood immediately available prior to chest tube insertion. Autotransfusion may be used.

PNEUMOMEDIASTINUM

A pneumomediastinum occurs when there is an accumulation of air in the mediastinal (middle) area of the chest cavity. It can occur after a trauma, or following a pneumothorax. It may also be referred to as mediastinal emphysema.

Patients with pneumomediastinum may show only mild or even no symptoms initially. However, symptoms will gradually worsen depending upon the amount of air in the chest cavity. Subcutaneous emphysema (palpated as "crepitus" – the popping and crackling sensation of air moving about in a tissue space) may be present around the trauma site. The patient may complain of chest pain that worsens during inspiration. The patient may also experience a sudden drop in oxygen saturation. Hamman's sign (a crunching sound that can be heard with each heart beat) may also be present.

DIAGNOSIS AND TREATMENT

Pneumomediastinum is primarily diagnosed by visualizing the presence of air in the chest, typically through a chest X-ray or computed tomography (CT) image.

In some cases, no treatment is required, as a small amount of air can be reabsorbed by the body through the mediastinal tissues. However, if the patient becomes hypotensive, as a result of pressure placed on the heart or surrounding vessels, a mediastinoscopy may be performed for a more complete evaluation and removal of the accumulated air. Another way to treat a pneumomediastinum would be to place a tube near the air leak through which to draw away the accumulated air and fluid.

A chest tube may be placed if the pneumomediastinum expands into a pneumothorax and complicates overall pulmonary function.

PNEUMOPERICARDIUM

Pneumopericardium is the presence of air in the pericardial sac surrounding the heart. Though a pneumopericardium can be congenital, it most often the result of a traumatic injury that occurs both in the lung and the pericardium. A pneumopericardium can also occur as the result of a puncture during a central line insertion. However, because the pericardium is thick and fibrous, such occurrences are rare.

Signs and symptoms of pneumopericardium include sudden onset chest pain, shortness of breath, cyanosis, and a dry cough. A pleural friction rub may be auscultated. The patient may also have Hamman's sign, which is a rasping sound on auscultation that occurs with the heart beat.

PULMONARY HYPERTENSION

Pulmonary hypertension is an abnormally elevated vascular pressure in the pulmonary artery. Patients with pulmonary hypertension typically have a resting mean pulmonary artery pressure greater than 25 mm Hg.

The elevated pressure usually results from changes within the pulmonary artery, the pulmonary vein, or the capillaries within the lungs. As a result, the right heart requires more effort to pump blood to the lungs. Right-side heart failure will eventually occur when blood becomes backed up within the circulatory system. The patient will then experience shortness of breath and increasing exercise intolerance as their pulmonary hypertension worsens.

SIGNS AND SYMPTOMS

The most common symptom of pulmonary hypertension is dyspnea as a result of decreased circulation to the lungs. The patient may also complain of fatigue or dizziness. Over time, exercise intolerance will become more pronounced, and the patient may complain of chest pain during increased activity as a result of greater cardiac effort to meet oxygenation demands. The patient may also have an elevated respiration rate, even during periods of rest.

As pulmonary hypertension worsens, the patient will also show signs of right-side heart failure. This includes peripheral edema, jugular venous distension, crackles in the lungs on auscultation, and hepatomegaly.

PRIMARY AND SECONDARY PULMONARY HYPERTENSION

Secondary pulmonary hypertension occurs when another disease process increases the pressure within the pulmonary artery. It typically occurs as a result of chronic lung diseases such as emphysema and chronic obstructive pulmonary disease (COPD). It may also have an underlying cardiac cause, such as left-side heart failure. Secondary pulmonary hypertension occurs most commonly in the older adult patient population.

Primary pulmonary hypertension is also referred to as idiopathic pulmonary hypertension, as it has no clear physiological cause. There is some indication that it may occur as a result of a genetic disorder. Primary pulmonary hypertension is more aggressive than secondary pulmonary hypertension, and typically affects younger patient populations.

DIAGNOSIS

There are a number of noninvasive tests that may be used to diagnose pulmonary hypertension. A patient with pulmonary hypertension may have ECG changes, such as peaked P waves and a bundle branch block. A chest X-ray may show cardiac changes associated with pulmonary hypertension, such as hypertrophy of the right ventricle. During an echocardiogram, pulmonary pressure can be estimated, and structural changes to the right side of heart can be visualized.

The most accurate way of diagnosing pulmonary hypertension is through a right-side cardiac catheterization. During the procedure, pulmonary pressures can be measured directly upon introduction of a catheter tip into the pulmonary arteries. Cardiac output can also be measured to determine the extent of right heart failure.

TREATMENT

The primary goal in treating pulmonary hypertension is to identify and treat the underlying cause of the elevated pressure in the pulmonary artery. The patient may be placed on adjunctive oxygen if the pulmonary hypertension is caused by chronic lung problems.

If a pulmonary embolism has caused the pulmonary hypertension, the patient may be placed on medications to help dissolve the clot, as well as starting anticoagulation therapy to prevent the development of future blood clots. The patient may also be treated surgically, by performing a thromboendarterectomy to remove any thrombus that has formed within the pulmonary artery.

If the cause of pulmonary hypertension is idiopathic, the patient may be prescribed medications that will directly dilate the pulmonary artery itself, such as prostacyclin (Epoprostenol), sildenafil (Revatio), or treprostinil (Remodulin).

Medications used to treat elevated pressure in the pulmonary artery include calcium channel blockers, Cardene, and Cardizem. Cardiac preload dysfunction may also be reduced using diuretics.

If the patient does not respond to other treatments, a lung transplant may be considered.

TEACHING FOR PATIENTS

A new diagnosis of pulmonary hypertension carries an average survival rate of about 3 years, if left untreated. The cause of death for patients with pulmonary hypertension is typically right-side heart failure. Therefore, it is vital that the patient be compliant with their therapy to ensure a good outcome. The patient should be taught to closely regulate their activities to avoid putting undue stress on their heart. The patient should be encouraged to eat foods that are low in sodium and cholesterol, and to restrict their fluid intake. Smoking cessation should also be recommended. The patient should be encouraged to accept the annual flu and pneumonia vaccines.

COR PULMONALE

With cor pulmonale, changes will gradually develop within the right ventricle as a result of chronically increased pressure in the pulmonary artery or the lungs. Cor pulmonale typically develops over time as a result of pulmonary hypertension, but it can also occur as a result of alveolar hypoxemia and emphysema. Acute cor pulmonale can also occur in cases of massive pulmonary embolism and acute respiratory distress syndrome (ARDS).

As a result of increased pressure within the lungs, the right ventricle undergoes structural changes to compensate for the increased afterload. With chronic cor pulmonale, ventricular hypertrophy takes place as a result of constant right ventricular hypertrophy. There is also a septal displacement toward the left ventricle, decreasing the cardiac output. Right ventricular dilation tends to predominate in cases of acute cor pulmonale.

SIGNS AND SYMPTOMS

Patients who present with cor pulmonale show signs and symptoms consistent with right-side heart failure and an underlying lung disease.

Patients may present with a 'barrel chest', and have crackles or wheezes on auscultation. In cases of COPD, hyperresonance may be heard on percussion. They may have increasing activity intolerance, and/or shortness of breath while at rest.

Signs and symptoms of right-side heart failure also include a cardiac murmur, and extra heart sounds such as an S3 or S4 sound irregularities. Further, the patient may have abnormal breath sounds on auscultation, jugular-venous distension, hepatomegaly, and/or peripheral edema.

TESTS USED TO DIAGNOSE COR PULMONALE

There are a number of tests available that can be utilized to diagnose cor pulmonale. A b-type natriuretic peptide (BNP) level can be drawn to assess the degree of cardiac muscle 'stretch' or dilation that occurs as a result of fluid overload. An arterial blood gas (ABG) can also be drawn to assess the patient's oxygenation level.

Cardiomegaly can be visualized directly using a chest X-ray. A V/Q scan can be done to rule out pulmonary embolism. On an echocardiogram, right ventricular hypertrophy and a septal shift can also be visualized, which may indicate cor pulmonale. Pressures within the pulmonary artery and right ventricle can also be checked directly using a cardiac catheterization procedure.

TREATMENT

Treatment for cor pulmonale focuses on the dual tasks of treating the right ventricular failure and the underlying lung disorder.

In treating the right ventricular failure, the patient will be prescribed diuretics to decrease cardiac preload burdens. Cardiac glycosides, such as digitalis, may also be prescribed to improve cardiac output by improving contractility.

Pulmonary treatment options differ depending upon the underlying cause of a lung disorder. Theophylline may be prescribed as a bronchodilator to treat COPD. Adjunctive oxygen may also be prescribed to treat COPD. In cases of pulmonary hypertension, patients may be prescribed Coumadin to treat frequent pulmonary embolism. Phosphodiesterase inhibitors such as sildenafil or tadalafil may be prescribed to treat primary pulmonary hypertension.

VENTILATOR-ASSOCIATED PNEUMONIA

Ventilator-associated pneumonia (VAP) is defined as a lung infection that occurs after a patient has been breathing with the assistance of a mechanical ventilator for more than 48 hours. Pseudomonas is the microorganism typically responsible for causing VAP. Patients on the ventilator are at greater risk for acquiring pneumonia because an endotracheal (ET) tube is inserted deeply into the pulmonary passages, and thus bypasses many of the natural immune defenses of the lungs. VAP places an inordinate amount of stress upon a critically ill patient's immune system, resulting in a high risk for mortality. Thus, diligent care should be taken to prevent the occurrence of VAP.

SIGNS AND SYMPTOMS

The most common sign of the ventilator-associated pneumonia (VAP) is the presence of a low-grade fever that occurs as a systemic immune response. Conversely, some patients may experience a subnormal body temperature. The presence of thick, purulent sputum may be an indicator of VAP, as well. The patient may also experience hypoxia and low oxygen saturation levels as a result of alveolar inflammation.

New infiltrates on a chest X-ray indicate the presence of accumulating fluid or secretions, and should be investigated. An elevated white-blood cell count will indicate the presence of an infection. Blood cultures and sputum specimens will identify the microorganism that is causing the pneumonia, and sensitivity testing can help identify the most effective antibiotic to use in treatment.

RISK FACTORS FOR DEVELOPING VENTILATOR-ASSOCIATED PNEUMONIA

Patients who are at risk for developing ventilator-associated pneumonia (VAP) are those that have been on a mechanical ventilator for an extended period of time – at a minimum, more than 48 hours, which is the baseline incubation period for any bacteria introduced via the ventilation process (as differentiated from an infection already developing prior to the time of intubation). Because poor nutrition can decrease the effectiveness of the body's immune system, patients who are not receiving adequate nutrition are also at increased risk for developing VAP. VAP is prevalent in elderly patients, and patients with a previous diagnosis of lung disease are also at increased risk. Patients who lay in a supine position rather than with the head of the bed elevated are at risk of developing VAP secondary to the aspiration of gastric secretions.

PREVENTION

Because ventilator-associated pneumonia (VAP) carries a high risk of mortality and substantial treatment costs as well, there is a significant focus on prevention. Standard infection control precautions should be closely observed, including hand washing both before and between patient care activities. A closed suctioning system should be utilized, and care should be taken to prevent the collection of humidification in the tubing. The head of the patient's bed should be maintained at a 30-degree angle, and the endotracheal tube cuff should be kept inflated to prevent aspiration of stomach secretions. Proper oral care and suctioning should be performed regularly to prevent accumulation of microorganisms in the mouth. If the patient is going to be intubated for an extended period of time, tracheostomy placement should be considered.

TREATMENT

Once the microorganism responsible for triggering the ventilator-associated pneumonia (VAP) is identified, antibiotics will be prescribed to treat the infection. These may include Cefepime, Vancomycin, or Ciprofloxacin. If the patient maintains a temperature greater than 101.5 degrees Fahrenheit, antipyretics may also be prescribed. If the patient has copious secretions, they may require percussion treatment to ease expectoration. The patient's heart rate, blood pressure, oxygen saturation, and fluid status should be closely monitored. Appropriate nutrition (e.g., tube feeding or TPN) should be administered, as it helps to bolster the immune system. If prolonged intubation is required to support the patient's oxygen needs, a tracheotomy may be necessary.

BAROTRAUMAS AND VOLUTRAUMA

Barotrauma and volutrauma are ventilator induced lung injuries, both of which can lead to the development of acute respiratory distress syndrome (ARDS). Barotrauma is a lung injury that results from a high level of gaseous pressure, such as that produced by the mechanical ventilator. It can be prevented by placing the patient on a tidal volume that meets but does not exceed the patient's respiratory needs.

Volutrauma is lung injury that results from either overextension or under-inflation of the lung. Lowering peak inspiratory pressures by, for example, decreasing the tidal volume, can help prevent overextension. Under-inflation can be prevented by placing the patient on a positive end-expiratory pressure (PEEP) mode to help keep the alveoli open.

SLEEP APNEA

OBSTRUCTIVE SLEEP APNEA

Obstructive sleep apnea results from passive collapse of the pharynx during sleep, often associated with narrow or restricted upper airway (micrognathia, obesity, enlarged tonsils). It is most common in middle-aged overweight males and is exacerbated by drinking and ingesting alcohol or sedative drugs before sleeping. Symptoms include daytime somnolence, headache, cognitive impairment, depression, personality changes, recent increase in weight, and impotence. Patients often snore loudly with cycles of breath cessation caused by apneic periods up to 60 seconds, occurring at least 30 times a night despite continued chest wall and abdominal movements, indicating automatic attempt to breathe. ECG changes may indicate bradydysrhythmia during apnea and tachydysrhythmia when breathing resumes. Nocturnal polysomnography shows apneic periods >10 seconds (usually 20-40 seconds). There may be hypopnea with reduction of airflow. Both apneic and hypopneic periods result in reduced oxyhemoglobin saturation. If condition is severe, hypoxemia or hypercarbia may persist during waking hours.

CENTRAL SLEEP APNEA AND CENTRAL ALVEOLAR HYPOVENTILATION SYNDROME

Central sleep apnea involves apneic and hypopneic episodes without obstruction and usually results from cardiac or neurological disorders that cause impairment of ventilation. Snoring is usually mild, and individuals may complain of insomnia because they awaken frequently. Chest wall and abdominal movements do not occur during apneic periods with this breathing-related sleep disorder. Cheyne-Stokes respirations may be present (apnea, 10 to 60 seconds of hyperventilation, followed by another period of apnea). Nocturnal polysomnography shows decreased respiratory effort associated with decreased oxygen saturation.

Central alveolar hypoventilation syndrome results from impaired ventilatory control, characterized by low arterial oxygen levels and hypoventilation without apnea or hypopnea. Hypoventilation periods may persist for several minutes with sustained arterial oxygen desaturation and increased levels of carbon dioxide. This condition is often associated with obesity.

Individual may complain of feeling excessively sleep or having insomnia. If condition is severe, hypoxemia or hypercarbia may persist during waking hours.

CONSERVATIVE THERAPEUTIC INTERVENTIONS FOR SLEEP APNEA

Sleep apnea intervention usually includes CPAP although surgery may also be recommended as a last resort. However, intervention usually begins by eliminating those factors that may influence the condition. In mild cases, conservative intervention alone may be sufficient:

- Avoid drinking any alcohol in the evening as it may increase sleep apnea.
- Stop smoking as it impairs airways.
- Treat allergies, which may cause swelling and obstruction of airways.
- Control obesity by diet and exercise.
- Avoid night shift work if possible.
- Review medications with physician as some (such as tranquilizers and short acting β-blockers) may increase apnea, especially if taken in the evening.
- Change sleep position if polysomnography indicates OSA occurs only in one position (such as while supine) although this alone is usually not sufficient treatment for most people as it can be difficult to control sleep position even with bolsters and pillows.
- Bariatric surgery may be recommended if the patient is unable to lose weight and obesity is severely compromising respirations/ventilation.

THERAPEUTIC INTERVENTIONS

Potential therapies for sleep disorders include:

CPAP	Education regarding the continuous positive airway pressure (CPAP) devices should include the different types of masks available and the differences in the types of machines available: Bi-level PAP: Changes pressure during exhalation to facilitate breathing. AutoPap/APAP: Has adjustable pressure rather than fixed. The patient should understand the importance of using a humidifier to prevent drying of mucous membranes and should understand that using the CPAP is not an option or a temporary or part-time solution but should be used with every sleep, whether at night or while napping during the daytime.
Oral/ dental devices	Some patients with mild sleep apnea may be prescribed oral or dental devices, which fit inside the mouth or are fastened around the head to open the airway during sleep. Devices include: Mandibular repositioning device. Tongue retaining device. Patients should be cautioned to have devices fitted by professionals, such as a dentist, in order to avoid damage to the teeth, mouth, or jaw.

Monitoring and Diagnostics

ABG

An arterial blood gas (ABG) sample is drawn to assess the patient's oxygenation status. It is obtained by drawing blood from an artery to assess the patient's pH, partial pressures of carbon dioxide and oxygen, oxygen saturations, and bicarbonate level. During an ABG, the patient's lactate, hemoglobin, and a number of electrolytes can be assessed as well. The blood is most typically drawn from the radial artery because it carries the least chance of occluding and can be easily compressed after the blood is obtained. However, arterial blood can also be drawn from the brachial or femoral arteries.

INDICATION

An ABG is indicated to assess the patient's cellular oxygenation status, particularly if they are presenting with symptoms of severe respiratory distress in cases of asthma, chronic obstructive pulmonary disease (COPD), or pulmonary embolism. It may also be obtained to assess the effectiveness of therapies such as BiPAP or mechanical ventilation. An ABG is typically obtained 1 to 2 hours after initiating BiPAP or mechanical ventilation, and the settings are adjusted accordingly. An ABG may also be obtained to assess the patient's acid-base level in certain chronic conditions such as diabetes, sleep apnea, heart failure, or kidney failure.

DRAWING ABG SAMPLES

Prior to the start of the test the procedure should be explained to the patient, including the risks and benefits of performing the test. An arterial blood gas (ABG) sample can be drawn from the radial, brachial, or femoral arteries. If the radial artery is the site chosen from which to obtain the ABG sample, an Allen's test should be performed to ensure adequate collateral circulation to the hand. The radial pulse should be palpated, taking care not to obliterate it. Once the pulse has been located, the site should be cleansed with Betadine and/or alcohol. The needle should then be inserted into the wrist at a 45-degree angle. Obtain 3 ccs of arterial blood before withdrawing the needle. Hold pressure on the artery at the puncture site. Ensure that there are no air bubbles in the syringe, as they may dissolve into the blood and create a falsely elevated result.

ALLEN'S TEST

An Allen's test is performed to test the patient's collateral circulation prior to drawing an arterial blood gas (ABG). Before starting the test, the patient should elevate their hand and make a fist for 20 to 30 seconds. The radial and ulnar arteries are then manually occluded. When the patient's opens their hand, blanching should be noted on the palm and fingernails. When pressure on the ulnar artery is released, color should return to the patient's hand within 7 to 10 seconds. If color does not return to the patient's hand, it indicates the patient's ulnar circulation is insufficient to provide adequate collateral circulation if occlusion of the radial artery occurs as a complication of the needle insertion to obtain the ABG sample. This means that the patient at increased risk for ischemia within the hand. If the patient fails the Allen's test, another site should be chosen for drawing an ABG sample.

ABG TESTS

The pH determines if the patient's blood sample is acidic or alkalotic. The normal range for pH is 7.35 to 7.45. If the pH is less than 7.35, the patient is in acidosis. If the pH is greater than 7.45, the patient is in alkalosis.

PO_2 measures the partial pressure of oxygen that is dissolved in the blood. The normal range of PO_2 is 90 to 100 mmHg.

PCO_2 measures the partial pressure of carbon dioxide. It indicates the effectiveness of that patient's ventilation. An abnormally high PCO_2 indicates hypoventilation, while an abnormally low PCO_2 indicates hyperventilation. The normal range for PCO_2 is 35 to 45 mmHg.

Bicarbonate (HCO_3) is an alkaline solution that is produced by the kidneys to help regulate pH. The normal range for HCO_3 is 22 to 26 mEq/L.

ABG TEST RESULTS

Begin by looking at the pH. If the patient's pH is less than 7.35, they are in acidosis. If the pH is greater than 7.45, they are in alkalosis. Next, look at the patient's carbon dioxide level (PCO_2). If the PCO_2 level is less than 35 mmHg, the patient is in respiratory alkalosis. If the patient's PCO_2 is greater than 45 mmHg, they are in respiratory acidosis. Finally, look at the patient's bicarbonate (HCO_3) level. If the patient's HCO_3 level is less than 22 mEq/L, the patient is in metabolic acidosis. If the patient's HCO_3 is greater than 26 mEq/L, the patient is in metabolic alkalosis.

RESPIRATORY ACIDOSIS

In respiratory acidosis the patient has an elevated carbon dioxide (CO_2) level that occurs as a result of hypoventilation. CO_2 is an acidic waste product that is eliminated from the body during exhalation. Hypoventilation causes inadequate CO_2 elimination, which results in a rising CO_2 level within the blood. Respiratory acidosis is caused by any condition that impedes the respiratory drive, such as a drug overdose, abdominal distention, chest wall injury, respiratory arrest, or emphysema.

Rising levels of CO_2 secondarily result in central nervous system depression. The patient may then show symptoms of a decreased level of consciousness, lethargy, headaches, muscle weakness, and tremors. The patient may also experience hypotension, tachycardia, or tachyarrhythmias.

METABOLIC ACIDOSIS

Metabolic acidosis is caused by either an increase of the acidic components within the body, or by a decrease in the basic components available within the body. An increase of the body's acid level (acidemia) can be caused by renal failure or by hypoaldosteronism. The acidic level can also be elevated in cases of ketoacidosis secondary to starvation or diabetes, or by lactic acidosis. A loss of base components within the body can be caused by chronic diarrhea or as the result of a pancreatic or biliary fistula.

Patients who are in metabolic acidosis may experience nausea, vomiting, hyperventilation, and central nervous system depression. Severe metabolic acidosis may lead to seizures, coma, or life-threatening ventricular dysrhythmias.

RESPIRATORY ALKALOSIS

Respiratory alkalosis is caused by hyperventilation, causing too much CO_2 to be eliminated from the bloodstream. It can be caused by a rapid respiratory rate secondary to hypoxemia or anxiety. Pulmonary disorders such as pneumonia or pulmonary embolism may also cause respiratory alkalosis. Other causes include pain, sepsis, hepatic insufficiency, and acute myocardial infarction, as well as central nervous system disorders such as cerebral vascular accident and trauma.

Patients in respiratory alkalosis may experience agitation and syncope, and may complain of tingling in their extremities. Severe respiratory alkalosis may lead to seizures, cardiac dysrhythmias, and tetany.

METABOLIC ALKALOSIS

Metabolic alkalosis is typically caused by a loss of fixed acids within the body, or by an increase in the level of buffer in the blood. Loss of fixed acids can occur as a result of aggressive diuresis, vomiting, and frequent gastric suctioning. An elevated buffer within the blood can be caused by excessive ingestion of baking soda, large quantity blood transfusions, or by administration of large amounts of sodium bicarbonate, lactate, or acetate.

Patients experiencing metabolic alkalosis may complain of dizziness, nausea, vomiting, and diarrhea. They may also experience seizures, cardiac dysrhythmias secondary to hypokalemia, confusion, and hypoventilation.

DETERMINING ACID-BASE COMPENSATION

Acid-base compensation is performed by the body in an attempt to correct an acid-base disorder and return the blood to a normal pH level. First, determine the primary cause of the acid-base disorder. If the pH is acidotic, determine if the cause is from metabolic acidosis or respiratory acidosis. Conversely, if the pH is alkalotic, determine if the cause is respiratory alkalosis or metabolic alkalosis.

To determine the adequacy of compensation, consider the patient's pH, HCO_3 and PCO_2. Compensation has not occurred if the pH and PCO_2, or the pH and HCO_3 levels, are abnormal. Partial compensation has occurred if the pH, HCO_3 and PCO_2 are abnormal. Complete compensation has occurred when the pH is normal, even if the HCO_3 and PCO_2 levels remain abnormal.

DETERMINING PATIENT'S LEVEL OF OXYGENATION

A patient's level of oxygenation is determined by checking their partial pressure of oxygen (PaO_2) and their hemoglobin oxygen saturation (SaO_2). PaO_2 refers to how effectively oxygen is able to move from the lungs into the bloodstream. SaO_2 refers to the percentage of hemoglobin that is completely saturated with oxygen, and is dependent upon a normal PaO_2 to maintain normal levels. The normal range for PaO_2 is between 90 to 100 mmHg. When the patient's PaO_2 is between 60 and 80 mmHg, the patient is considered to be mildly hypoxemic. When the patient's PaO_2 is between 40 and 60 mmHg, they are considered to be moderately hypoxemic. Severe hypoxemia occurs when the patient's PaO_2 is less than 40 mmHg. Adjunctive oxygen should be administered for a PaO_2 less than 60 mmHg. Immediate intervention is required for a PaO_2 less than 26 mmHg, as death is imminent.

ARTERIAL OXYGEN SATURATION AND VENOUS OXYGEN SATURATION

Arterial oxygen saturation (SaO_2) measures the amount of oxygen that is bound to hemoglobin and dissolved in plasma in arterial blood. It measures the degree of oxygenation produced by the lungs. A normal SaO_2 range is 90 to 100%. SaO_2 can be measured with a pulse oximeter probe (abbreviated SpO_2) or by drawing an arterial blood gas sample.

Venous oxygen saturations (SvO_2) measure the amount of oxygen bound to hemoglobin and dissolved within the plasma of the blood when it is returning from the body to the heart and lungs. SvO_2 measures cardiac output and tissue oxygen consumption. The normal range for SvO_2 is between 60 and 80%.

VENOUS GAS

Venous oxygen saturation (SvO_2) is measured by drawing a mixed venous gas sample from the distal port of the pulmonary artery catheter. Drawing blood from the distal port provides a sampling of blood from different parts of the body prior to be being oxygenated by the lungs. Mixed venous blood can be drawn intermittently and assessed by being sent to the lab, or it can be monitored continuously using a fiberoptic attachment on the distal tip of the catheter.

The normal range for SvO_2 is 60 to 80%, which indicates adequate cardiac output and tissue perfusion. An SvO_2 between 40 and 60% indicates inadequate tissue oxygenation. An SvO_2 less than 40% indicates a significant oxygen supply-demand imbalance; either the cardiac output is inadequate, or tissue oxygen demands are elevated.

PULSE OXIMETRY

Pulse oximetry can be initiated by placing a pulse oximeter probe on a thin portion of a patient's anatomy, such as over a fingertip or an earlobe. When connected to a monitor, a light on one end of the probe comes on. It emits red and infrared waves to the other side of the probe. The pulse oximeter then measures the amount of oxygen bound to the hemoglobin, taking into account the fact that hemoglobin with less oxygen bound to it is darker in color than hemoglobin that is replete with oxygen. That measurement is then calculated as the patient's SpO_2.

RELIABILITY OF MONITORING

Care should be taken in monitoring pulse oximetry, as a number of factors can interfere with the accuracy of the results. Decreased arterial flow secondary to hypothermia or hypotension can result in ineffective pulse oximetry. Anemia may cause an inaccurate SpO_2 value, as can hyperlipidemia.

If the patient's venous pressure is elevated, the patient's SpO_2 may be inaccurate. If the patient's SpO_2 is inaccurate and does not match the patient's clinical picture, it may be the result of technical factors, such as motion artifact. Strong ambient light may also cause interference in SpO_2 monitoring.

NURSING INTERVENTIONS

The patient's oxygen saturation should be assessed and charted along with their vital signs. A general respiratory assessment should be completed and the plethysmographic (pleth) waveform should be assessed to ensure that perfusion is adequate. If the pleth is poor, the patient's clinical picture should be further assessed to see if the problem is due to the patient's medical status or arising from equipment difficulties. A poor pleth might be the result of cool extremities, or a loose lead connection. Timely troubleshooting should be undertaken to ensure that all equipment is properly functioning. The pulse oximetry probe placement should be rotated to prevent tissue breakdown, and frequent skin care around the probe should be performed.

END-TIDAL CO$_2$

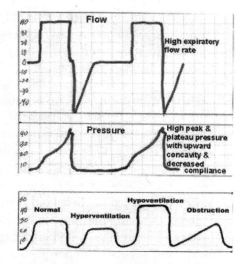

End-tidal carbon dioxide (ETCO$_2$), which is the partial pressure or concentration of carbon dioxide at the end of expiration, is measured by capnography through mainstream or sidestream sampling. Normal values are 5% to 6%, which corresponds to 35 to 45 mm Hg. ETCO$_2$ often correlates with PaCO$_2$ within 1.0 mm Hg with stable ventilation and perfusion, so ETCO$_2$ can sometimes be used to estimate PaCO$_2$ but should not be relied on as it may be imprecise. The waveform is monitored to assess respiratory function. With the normal waveform, the line rises with exhalation, levels and drops with inhalation. The point immediately before the drop (the end point of exhalation) is where $ETCO_2$ is measured. Hyperventilation lowers the waveform and increases the number of waveforms while hypoventilation raises the waveform but decreases the number. A "shark fin" sloped waveform (plateau is lost) indicates obstruction, such as may occur with asthma, COPD, or bronchospasm.

CONDITIONS THAT INCREASE ETCO₂

$ETCO_2$ is monitored to ensure that the lungs are ventilated and that the mask or endotracheal tube is correctly positioned, to estimate the $PaCO_2$, and to identify changes in pulmonary blood flow or dead space ventilation:

- Conditions that increase $ETCO_2$ include those that result in increased production of CO_2, such as high fever, sepsis, seizures, increased metabolic rate, and increased cardiac output. With return of spontaneous circulation after cardiac arrest, the $ETCO_2$ level may increase suddenly because of CO_2 washout.
- Conditions that decrease ventilation at the level of the alveoli also result in increased $ETCO_2$, including COPD, hypoventilation, muscle weakness/paralysis (muscular dystrophy, spinal cord injury), and depression of the respiratory center of the brain. Hypoventilation (characterized by $ETCO_2$ greater than 45 mm Hg) may result from head trauma, sedation, stroke, drug overdose, and inebriation.
- Additionally, $ETCO_2$ may increase because of malfunction of equipment or setting of incorrect parameters, including patient rebreathing, ventilator circuit leaks, and exhausted CO_2 absorbers.

CONDITIONS THAT DECREASE ETCO₂

$ETCO_2$ can be affected by many different factors. Those factors that result in decreased $ETCO_2$ include:

- Conditions that decrease production of CO_2 so that less is delivered to the lungs and expired include hypothermia, pulmonary hypoperfusion, decreased cardiac output, hemorrhage, shock, pulmonary embolism, hypovolemia, and hypertension. Patients undergoing CPR for cardiac arrest are unlikely to survive if $ETCO_2$ level is ≤10 mm Hg after 20 minutes of resuscitation attempts.
- Decreased $ETCO_2$ may also result from hyperventilation: Hyperventilation (characterized by $ETCO_2$ less than 35 mm Hg) may occur with cardiac arrest, hypotension, and marked pulmonary edema.
- $ETCO_2$ may also decrease because of malfunction of equipment or setting of incorrect parameters, including disconnection of some part of the ventilator, intubation into the esophagus rather than the trachea, obstruction of the airway, leak about the cuff of the endotracheal tube, and poor sampling technique.

Note: intubation into the esophagus generally elicits very low $ETCO_2$ results, but if the patient had ingested carbonated beverages or antacids, the levels may be artificially increased.

Non-Invasive Positive Pressure Ventilation

CPAP

Continuous positive airway pressure (CPAP) is provided through a device that is prescribed for patients who have been diagnosed with obstructive sleep apnea (OSA). In OSA, the soft tissue of the throat relaxes and partially collapses during sleep, causing periods of apnea. This increases the patient's risk for heart attack or stroke, secondary to inadequate oxygenation. Wearing a CPAP mask at night creates positive pressure throughout the respiratory cycle, keeping the airway open while the patient is sleeping. It typically results in improved sleep quality, and decreases the risk of health problems associated with OSA.

BiPAP

"BiPAP" or Bi-level Positive Airway Pressure is provided through a device that provides positive pressure on two levels. First, "Inspiratory Positive Airway Pressure" (IPAP) is delivered to decrease pulmonary workload by providing pressurized air to the lungs during inspiration. Second, "Expiratory Positive Airway Pressure" (EPAP) is given to sustain alveolar expansion during expiration. As a result, the patient's functional reserve capacity is increased.

BiPAP is indicated for patients who have elevated carbon dioxide levels secondary to chronic obstructive pulmonary disease, pulmonary edema, pneumonia, or congestive heart failure. It is preferred over mechanical ventilation if the cause of the impaired gas exchange is easily reversible.

NON-INVASIVE POSITIVE PRESSURE DEVICES

Non-invasive positive pressure devices such as BiPAP are indicated for patients in acute respiratory distress with elevated carbon dioxide levels. This includes patients with pulmonary edema, asthma, chronic obstructive pulmonary disease, or congestive heart failure. It may also be prescribed to provide oxygen to patients who have failed extubation.

BiPAP should be used for patients who are having dyspnea with a respiratory rate greater than 25 breaths per minute. Physical findings, such as accessory muscle use or respiratory paradox, support the need for a noninvasive positive pressure device. BiPAP should be considered if the patient has a $PaCO_2$ greater than 45 mmHg, a pH between 7.10 and 7.35, or a PaO_2 less than 200 mmHg.

NURSING CONSIDERATIONS

The patient's vital signs should be closely monitored during noninvasive positive pressure therapy to ensure the patient's heart rate, respiration rate, and pulse oximetry remains within an appropriate range. An arterial blood gas should be checked 1 to 2 hours after initiating noninvasive positive pressure therapy to ensure the patient is receiving an appropriate amount of oxygen. The patient's level of comfort should be frequently assessed, and the patient should be appropriately medicated for pain or anxiety. Because noninvasive continuous positive pressure devices require a good seal to ensure effectiveness, the mask should be left in place until the patient's respiratory status improves. Until that time, the patient should be kept NPO to prevent aspiration and removal of the mask. If BiPAP is to be used for an extended period of time, regular oral care should also be provided.

CONTRAINDICATIONS

There are several contraindications that preclude the use of a noninvasive positive pressure device. First, the use of a noninvasive positive pressure device would be ineffective on a patient who is uncooperative, cognitively impaired, or agitated. Because positive pressure masks require a good seal to be effective, the patient must be cooperative in keeping the mask in place for the therapy to be effective. Patients with increased secretions or a high risk for aspiration should not be placed on a noninvasive positive pressure device because it increases the risk for pneumonia and other complications. Patients who have had a recent myocardial infarction or gastrointestinal surgery should not be placed on BiPAP because it alters the intrathoracic pressure. Noninvasive positive pressure devices are also contraindicated in patients who have had recent facial trauma or surgery, as the mask may cause further facial damage.

Mechanical Ventilation

Mechanical ventilation is provided for patients whose breathing is inadequate to sustain life. It is indicated for respiratory acidosis, tachypnea greater than 30 breaths per minute, a volume capacity less than 15 ml/kg, or a PaO_2 less than 55 mmHg. Respiratory conditions that might require mechanical ventilation include chronic obstructive pulmonary disease, acute respiratory distress syndrome, or respiratory arrest. Mechanical ventilation is also indicated to support a patient during collapse of other organ systems, such as in neuromuscular disease, spinal cord injury, hypotension secondary to sepsis, congestive heart failure, or shock.

> **Review Video: Medical Ventilators**
> Visit mometrix.com/academy and enter code: 679637

TIDAL VOLUME, RATE, SENSITIVITY, FiO₂ AND PEEP

Tidal volume refers to the volume of air given to the patient with each breath. Care must be taken in setting tidal volume, as too much can cause volutrauma, and too little can cause atelectasis. Tidal volume is prescribed based upon the patient's ideal body weight and height.

Rate refers to the minimum number of breaths per minute the patient is to receive. Sensitivity refers to the amount of negative pressure the patient must produce in order to trigger a breath above the control rate. FiO_2 is the amount of oxygen that is given to the patient with each breath. Initially, the FiO_2 is set at 100% (1.0), and gradually titrated down based upon the patient's needs.

Positive end-expiratory pressure refers to the amount of continued pressure exerted by the ventilator on the lungs in order to reduce alveolar closure during expiration.

WEANING USING SIMV AND PSV

There are three methods of withdrawing ventilator support. The first is using synchronous intermittent mandatory ventilation (SIMV). Weaning using SIMV is done by gradually decreasing the number of mandatory breaths per minute, allowing the patient to do more and more of the work of breathing. As long as the patient is able to tolerate the additional workload, the control rate is decreased by 2 breaths every 1 to 2 hours.

In pressure support ventilation (PSV), the patient initiates all breaths by themselves, and the ventilator provides enough pressure support to give the patient an adequate tidal volume. Weaning using PSV is done by gradually decreasing the amount of pressure supplied.

ASSIST-CONTROL AND SIMV

Assist-Control (AC) is the ventilator setting most commonly used after intubation. On an AC setting, the patient's respiratory control rate, tidal volume, sensitivity, FiO_2, and PEEP can be adjusted as necessary. On the AC setting, the ventilator provides breaths at a minimum control rate. However, if the patient attempts to initiate a breath independently, above the control rate, they are permitted to receive a set amount of tidal volume.

Synchronized intermittent mandatory ventilation (SIMV) was developed as a way to wean a patient from the ventilator by facilitating spontaneous breaths within the patient. SIMV has a set number of minimum breaths per minute, during which the patient receives the prescribed tidal volume. If the patient initiates a breath above the set rate, they are allowed to take in as much volume as they can, rather than receiving a pre-set tidal volume.

IMPACT OF MECHANICAL VENTILATION ON HEMODYNAMICS

The extent to which **positive pressure ventilation** (PPV) can positively impact hemodynamics depends on the pressure settings and the patient's underlying condition. With normal cardiac status, the body can usually compensate for any negative effects of PPV; and, in some cases, patients with underlying cardiac disease may benefit. For example, in patients with left ventricular heart failure, PPV decreases left ventricular afterload, and this reduced resistance results in increased cardiac output and left ventricular ejection fraction. However, the patient is at increased risk of left failure when PPV is discontinued. If hypoxic pulmonary vasoconstriction is present before PPV is initiated, the increased oxygen flow inhibits vasoconstriction, inflates collapsed alveoli, and may reverse respiratory acidosis, resulting in increased oxygenated blood reaching the heart and coronary arteries and improved cardiovascular function. PPV takes over the work of breathing so the patient expends less energy and oxygen consumption decreases, and this improves oxygen delivery to the rest of the body.

PEAK INSPIRATORY PRESSURE IN MECHANICAL VENTILATION

Peak inspiratory pressure (PIP) is the highest pressure delivered to the lungs and needed to overcome airway resistance and decreased pulmonary compliance in order to inflate alveoli in mechanical ventilation. PIP is measured at the end of the inspiratory phase. Management of PIP depends on the type of ventilation system:

- **Pressure control ventilation**: The PIP is set and remains constant throughout ventilation regardless of any changes in resistance or compliance. PIP is usually set at 20 to 25 cm H_2O and adjusted up or down by about 5 cm H_2O at a time in order to maintain tidal volume of 6-8 mL/Kg of ideal body weight. PIP should never be above 40 cm H_2O because of the risk of barotrauma and pneumothorax. PIP is usually about 10 cm H_2O greater than maximal plateau pressure.
- **Volume control ventilation**: The PIP will vary as needed to ensure stable tidal volume. PIP increases with increased peak inspiratory flow setting, PEEP, auto-PEEP, and tidal volume but decreases with lower descending ramp flow. PIP and plateau pressure also increase with decreased pulmonary compliance. High peak pressure and low plateau pressure indicates obstruction.

PLATEAU PRESSURE

Plateau pressure (Pplat) is measured with an inspiratory pause (usually 0.5-1.0 second) immediately after the peak inspiratory pressure (PIP) and the beginning of the expiratory flow. Plateau pressure represents the average pressure at the alveoli and small airways. Plateau pressure should be maintained at less than 30 cm H_2O to avoid risk of barotrauma. Normal plateau pressure is usually about 10 cm H_2O less than peak pressure. Changes in the plateau pressure:

- Increased PiP and increased Pplat (problem at small airways/alveoli): Tension pneumothorax, endobronchial intubation, deceased pulmonary compliance, pulmonary edema, pleural effusion, abdominal ascites, severe pneumonia, increased tidal volume.

- Increased PIP but stable Pplat (problem with airway requiring increased pressure to overcome): Obstructed/Twisted ET tube, airway obstruction, increased flow rate. With normal lung function, the plateau pressure is only slightly less than the peak pressure.

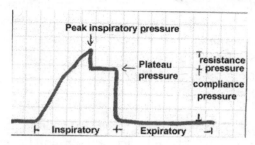

Note: with increased compliance, PIP and Pplat decrease; with decreased compliance, PIP and Pplat increase.

NORMAL MECHANICAL VENTILATION WAVEFORMS

Mechanical ventilation waveforms may vary from one manufacturer to another and from one setting to another. For example, with pressure-controlled ventilation, the pressure waveform will be consistent but the flow and volume waveforms may change. With volume-controlled ventilation, the volume waveform will be consistent but the pressure and flow waveforms may change. With all types of ventilators, there are three basic parameters commonly displayed: Pressure, volume, and flow.

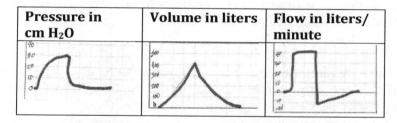

Pressure in cm H_2O	Volume in liters	Flow in liters/ minute

Inspiration is represented by the rising lines and plateaus and expiration by the falling and extended lines. The shape of the waveforms will change depending on the setting. The waveforms may help to identify the cause of an alarm and to detect air trapping, increased airway resistance, overdistention, and obstruction.

TYPES OF WAVEFORMS

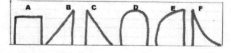

There are six different **types of waveforms** possible with displays of pressure, flow, and volume, depending on the settings:

- **A: Square** waveform indicates constant flow. For example, if a flowrate is set at 58 L/min, the flow will stay at that rate throughout the cycle.
- **B. Ascending/Accelerating ramp** indicates maximum flow at the end of inspiration.
- **C: Descending/Decelerating ramp** indicates maximum flow at the beginning of inspiration, reaching zero at the end.
- **D: Sinusoidal/Sine** indicates maximum flow/volume/pressure halfway through inspiration.

- **E: Exponential rising** indicates the greatest flow at the beginning and the least and the end.
- **F: Exponential decaying** indicates passive exhalation.

Pressure waveforms may include square, exponential rise, and sinusoidal. **Flow waveforms** may include square, ascending ramp, descending ramp, sinusoidal, and exponential decay. Both ascending ramp and sinusoidal flows may result in air hunger even though the slow flow allows more time for the gas to disperse throughout the lungs and may improve oxygenation. **Volume waveforms** may include ascending ramp and sinusoidal.

AIRWAY RESISTANCE

Airway resistance is the resistance of non-elastic forces in the lung to air flow, determined by the airway size and patency as well as airflow turbulence and obtained by subtracting the plateau pressure from the peak inspiratory pressure and dividing that by the airflow (usually 1/sec). Normal airway resistance is 2 to 5 cm H_2O/L/sec. A two-fold decrease in diameter of the airway results in a 16-fold increase in compliance. If the peak pressure is elevated but the plateau pressure stays the same, this indicates increased inspiratory airway resistance without increased inspiratory compliance. This may result from obstruction, such as from bronchospasm, secretions, kinking of ET tube, or condensation in the vent circuit. If however, the peak pressure and the plateau pressure both increase, this indicates decreased compliance, such as may occur with tension pneumothorax and overdistention. Patients with increased airway resistance (such as COPD patients) may need extended expiratory time. Ventilator corrections for increased airway resistance include: increasing inspiratory flow, increasing expiratory time, decreasing rate, or decreasing tidal volume. With increased PIP and stable Pplat, the tubing should be checked for kinks, patient suctioned for secretions, or bronchodilators administered for bronchospasm.

LUNG OVER-DISTENSION

Lung over-distention (AKA ventilator-induced lung injury) can result if the plateau pressure is greater than 30 cm H_2O. Over-distention is characterized by high expiratory flow rates and both high peak inspiratory pressure (PIP) and high plateau pressure (Pplat), as well as decreased compliance. The pressure waveform shows upward facing concavity, which indicates that compliance is worsening (Stress index >1). Over-distention of the alveoli may result in barotrauma. Over-distention may occur in regional areas of the lung when air under pressure flows more readily into healthy alveoli than damaged. High tidal volume may result in alveolar rupture. Utilizing lung-protective ventilation, such as low tidal volume, decreases risk of lung injury. When signs of over-distention occur, the pressure limit on the ventilator should be reduced and/or the tidal volume reduced. Generally, high volume, which results in stretching of the lung tissue, is more detrimental than increased airway pressure.

AIR TRAPPING

Air trapping (auto-PEEP) occurs with mechanical ventilation when the air that is inhaled is not completely exhaled so some remains "trapped" in the lungs because of decreased elasticity of the lung (elastic recoil) and increased expiratory airway resistance, resulting in barotrauma and hypotension. Patients with COPD and asthma are especially at risk of air trapping. Air trapping may impair venous return because of increased intrathoracic pressure, leading to cardiovascular collapse. To resolve air trapping, the inspiratory to expiratory ratio (I:E) must be decreased so that the expiratory time is extended, allowing time for the lungs to exhale the tidal volume. This can be achieved by various adjustments to the ventilator:

- Decrease tidal volume.
- Increase inspiratory gas flow
- Utilize a square waveform with full airflow from beginning to end of inspiration.

VENTILATOR ALARMS AND THEIR REMEDIES

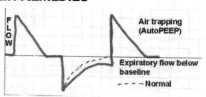

Ventilators contain a number of different alarms because failure of any of the ventilator functions may be life-threatening. **Ventilator alarms** include:

- **Power input:** Alarms warn if the power (electricity, pneumatic power) is shut off or a plug accidentally pulled to warm the nurse to check the power source. The alarm may also sound when battery power (for those with battery backup) is low.
- **Control circuit:** The alarm indicates that the control parameters are incorrectly set and must be reset or a problem exists in the control circuit, sometimes requiring a change in ventilator or maintenance.
- **Output**: Alarms indicate values are outside of expected parameters and settings may need to be adjusted. Output alarms may include:
  - Pressure: Assess ventilator for obstruction, circuit leak, malfunction and patient for obstruction, ET tube leak, and change in oxygenation.
  - Volume: Assess patient for possible leak about ET tube or disconnection from ventilator.
  - Flow: Assess patient for hyperventilation, apnea, or disconnection from ventilator.
  - Time: Assess patient for hyperventilation, apnea, and gas-trapping and ventilator for obstruction.
  - Inspired gas: Adjust gas temperature if high or low and FiO_2 if high or low.
  - Expired gas: Adjust as needed.

SBT

A "Spontaneous Breathing Trial" (SBT) is the preferred method for testing a patient's readiness for extubation. The SBT can be performed by removing the ventilator settings and placing the patient on either a T-piece trial or on CPAP. The patient should be closely monitored to ensure that they continue to achieve adequate oxygenation without becoming overworked. Blood pressure, respiration rate, heart rate, and arterial blood gases should be closely monitored. The SBT should last between 30 to 90 minutes. If the patient is able to support his or her own respiratory efforts during that time, extubation should be considered. If the patient fails the SBT (as indicated by poor oxygenation measures), they should be placed back on adequate ventilator settings, and weaning should continue until the patient is able to support their own respiratory needs.

> **Review Video: Ventilator Weaning**
> Visit mometrix.com/academy and enter code: 346956

WEANING AND EXTUBATION CRITERIA

Certain criteria should be fulfilled before ventilator weaning and extubation is initiated. The patient should be hemodynamically stable, and the underlying cause resulting in the need for mechanical ventilation should be resolved. Further, the patient should be able to protect their airway, have a strong cough, and be able to draw sufficient breaths to maintain adequate oxygenation without ventilator assistance.

Typical indicators that the patient is ready to be extubated include a spontaneous respiratory rate less than 25 breaths per minute and a tidal volume greater than 5 ml/kg. A PaO_2 greater than 200 mmHg or a negative inspiratory force (NIF) greater than 25 cm should also be considered.

NURSING CONSIDERATIONS FOR RECEIVING MECHANICAL VENTILATION

The patient's heart rate, blood pressure, and pulse oximetry should be carefully monitored while the patient is receiving mechanical ventilation to ensure an adequate oxygen supply. Arterial blood gases should be checked regularly to make sure the ventilator settings are fully meeting the patient's oxygenation needs. Sedation should be provided to ease pulmonary workload and to facilitate patient comfort. The head of the patient's bed should be elevated to at least 30 degrees to prevent aspiration of secretions. Frequent oral care and suctioning should be performed to prevent pneumonia. Nutrition should be provided to facilitate healing.

Pulmonary Pharmacology

DECONGESTANTS

Decongestants are medications prescribed to decrease mucosal secretions and inflammation. They work by stimulating the alpha-1 receptors within the lungs to cause vasoconstriction, thereby resulting in decreased congestion. This subsequently results in decreased airway resistance and decreased pulmonary workload. However, decongestants are contraindicated in patients with a past history of hypertension, as they may induce dangerously high blood pressure.

Medications classified as decongestants include Epinephrine, Phenylephrine, and Oxymetazoline. They can be given either as a nasal spray, directly applied to the mucous membranes, or as an oral medication.

BRONCHODILATORS

Bronchodilators are medications that cause the smooth muscle in the bronchi and bronchial tubes to dilate. This results in decreased pulmonary workload because airway resistance is decreased. Bronchodilators are most often prescribed to treat asthma and chronic obstructive pulmonary disease (COPD).

Bronchodilators are divided into three classifications: Short acting beta-2 agonists, long acting beta-2 agonists, and anticholinergics. Short acting beta-2 agonists provide immediate short-term relief from asthma symptoms. Medications included in this classification include Xopenex and Maxair. Long acting beta-2 agonists such as Advair and Symbicort take at least an hour before a full effect is obtained. However, both will provide bronchodilation over a period of twelve hours. Anticholinergics such as Ipratropium Bromide are often paired with a short acting beta-2 agonist to facilitate improved overall bronchodilation.

ANTIHISTAMINES

During an asthma attack, histamines are released in the body, causing vasodilation, bronchoconstriction, and inflammation within the lungs. Antihistamines are prescribed to target

116

the H_1 receptors located within the smooth muscle of the lungs, the endothelium, and the central nervous system, thereby causing vasoconstriction. This ultimately results in decreased inflammation and congestion. Common side effects of antihistamines include fatigue, blurred vision, dizziness, and gastrointestinal distress. Antihistamines are contraindicated in patients with a history of hypertension as they may induce a dangerously high blood pressure.

H_1 antihistamines include medications such as Diphenhydramine, Loratadine, Meclizine and Pheniramine.

Other Patient Care Problems

Endocrine

DIABETES MELLITUS

Diabetes is a disorder in which the pancreas is unable to produce an adequate amount of insulin, resulting in abnormally high blood sugar levels. Consistently elevated blood sugar levels can cause a myriad of complications among various body systems. Patients with uncontrolled diabetes have a significantly greater risk of experiencing a stroke or heart attack.

Patients with diabetes are divided into three groups. Those with Type I diabetes are unable to produce insulin, or don't produce enough insulin. Patients with type II diabetes are resistant to the insulin they do produce (rendering it ineffective), and they also produce an insufficient amount of insulin. Gestational diabetes occurs in women who are pregnant, but the symptoms typically resolve after the baby is delivered.

> **Review Video: <u>Diabetes Education: Health Belief Model</u>**
> Visit mometrix.com/academy and enter code: 954833

PATHOPHYSIOLOGY

Glucose is derived from the food a person eats, and is absorbed into the blood stream. The pancreas then secretes insulin in response to the elevated levels of glucose. The insulin stimulates the absorption of glucose into the cells to be broken down for energy. Insulin also controls to absorption of glucose into the liver for storage. The liver later releases the glucose into the bloodstream, as needed, in response to signs of hypoglycemia.

In diabetes, the patient may produce no insulin, or an insufficient amount of insulin, and may be resistant to the insulin that is produced. Without an adequate amount of insulin, the patient is unable to absorb the glucose, leaving it circulating in the blood stream until it is excreted by the kidneys.

DIAGNOSIS

There are a number of tests available to determine the level of glucose in a patient's blood. A fasting plasma glucose test is most commonly used to diagnose diabetes. The patient's blood is drawn after they have abstained from food and drink for 8 consecutive hours. A blood sugar level that is greater than 126 mg/dl is indicative of diabetes.

An oral glucose tolerance test is another way to diagnose diabetes. The patient's blood sugar is checked two hours after drinking a solution containing 75 grams of sugar. If their blood sugar climbs to greater than 200 mg/dl, the patient is suspected to have diabetes.

SIGNS AND SYMPTOMS

Type I diabetes is typically diagnosed during adolescence. Symptoms occur suddenly, and include nausea, vomiting, and dehydration. The patient may also experience diabetic ketoacidosis, in which the lack of insulin requires the body to burn muscle, fat, and liver cells for fuel. Increasing levels of the acidic ketone byproducts ultimately induce vomiting, dehydration, and confusion, and can lead to coma and death.

118

Type II diabetes is typically diagnosed in early to middle adulthood. Symptoms are gradual in onset, and may not be identified until the complications are pronounced.

Symptoms that occur in both Type I and Type II diabetes include fatigue, polydipsia (extreme thirst), polyphagia (extreme hunger), and polyuria (frequent urination). The patient may have poor wound healing as a result of their elevated blood sugar levels. The patient may also experience mental status changes, and sudden, unexplained weight loss.

COMPLICATIONS

Hyperglycemia, or elevated blood sugar levels, can lead to a large number of complications. The most significant of these complications occurs in the kidneys, in the nerves, and in the vasculature.

Patients with diabetes are at an increased risk for developing kidney failure as a result of damage to their kidneys. Kidney failure can lead to fluid overload, hypertension and subsequent heart failure.

Diabetes induced hyperglycemia can also cause nerve damage. The nerves of the autonomic nervous system are particularly sensitive to fluctuating blood sugar levels, and easily become damaged. The resulting neuropathies may leave the heart unable to properly regulate heart rate and blood pressure.

Diabetes also increases the rate at which the circulatory system develops atherosclerosis. This condition can ultimately place the patient at an increased risk for heart attack and stroke.

PREVENTION

The cause of diabetes is unknown. Although there is a strong genetic link, lifestyle choices have also been linked to the onset of diabetes. Factors such as hypertension, obesity, alcohol consumption, and a sedentary lifestyle have been shown to increase a person's risk for developing diabetes.

Controlling one's risk factors is the best way to prevent diabetes. The patient should be encouraged to perform regular exercise, and to maintain a diet that is low in sodium and fat. Alcohol consumption should be limited. If the patient has previously been diagnosed with hypertension, medication compliance should be encouraged to ensure appropriate blood pressure control.

TREATMENT

Because there is no cure for diabetes, the focus of treatment is to manage blood sugar levels to prevent further complications. The patient should monitor their blood sugar closely at home, and seek medical assistance if their blood sugar is below 60 mg/dl or greater than 400 mg/dl.

The patient should also be advised to make lifestyle changes to control their blood sugar levels. If the patient is obese, they should be encouraged to lose weight. The patient should also be taught to eat foods that are low in fat and carbohydrates, and high in fiber. Finally, the patient should be encouraged to limit their alcohol consumption, as it can lead to elevated blood sugar levels.

HEMOGLOBIN A1C TEST

Hemoglobin A1C is a test that determines if the patient's blood sugar level has been elevated over the past 120 days. Excess blood glucose attaches to hemoglobin, and hemoglobin containing red blood cells have a lifespan of approximately 120 days. A hemoglobin A1C test works by measuring the amount of glucose attached to the sampled red blood cells. It can be used to diagnose diabetes in conjunction with other testing, and it is helpful in determining the effectiveness of treatment. A hemoglobin A1c result greater than 8% indicates a consistently elevated blood sugar, meaning treatment should be altered for better blood sugar control.

MEDICATIONS TO CONTROL BLOOD SUGAR

Patients with mild cases of Type II diabetes may be able to control their blood sugar through diet and exercise. If they are unable to do so, an oral hypoglycemic agent such as metformin (Glucophage) or repaglinide (Prandin) may be prescribed to help lower blood sugar.

Most patients with Type I diabetes and some with Type II will be started on subcutaneous insulin injections to manage their blood sugar. Insulin therapy typically involves two types of insulin: a long acting insulin and a short acting insulin. Longer acting insulin, such as glargine (Lantus) and Ultralente work over a period of 18-36 hours for general management of blood sugar. Once an effective dosage has been determined, the patient typically takes the same dosage every day. Shorter acting insulin such as lispro (Humalog) and aspart (NovoLog) are typically taken with meals for short-term blood sugar management. The amount of insulin given is dependent on the patient's blood sugar prior to the start of the meal.

HYPERTENSION

Hypertension is a common condition in the United States. When combined with a diagnosis of diabetes, the patient's risk for heart attack and stroke increases dramatically. Blood pressure control is an important aspect of the prevention of other comorbidities related to hypertension and diabetes.

Angiotensin-converting enzyme (ACE) inhibitors are most commonly used to treat hypertension in patients with diabetes because they delay renal failure and reduce other complications. However, ACE inhibitors also create an increased risk of hypoglycemia. Therefore, diabetic patients taking ACE inhibitors should be taught to monitor their blood sugar particularly carefully. If they are unable to tolerate an ACE inhibitor, a beta-blocker or calcium channel blocker should be considered.

TEACHING FOR A PATIENT

The key to diabetes management is blood sugar control. In order to appropriately control their blood sugar, the patient should know when to check their blood sugar and how to provide treatment if it is outside the normal range. Patients with Type I diabetes should check their blood sugar before each meal and before they go to bed. Patients with Type II diabetes should check their blood sugar once a day, before breakfast. The patient's blood sugar should be between 90 and 130 mg/dl prior to eating. If it is too high or too low, the patient's treatment may need to be adjusted. The patients should also be taught to monitor their blood sugar closely during periods of illness or stress, as this may cause their glucose levels to become erratic.

If the patient is taking subcutaneous insulin, they should be taught how to administer injections. They should also be instructed about the importance of rotating injection sites to prevent creating scar tissue.

METABOLIC SYNDROME

Metabolic syndrome is a condition that includes 3 of 5 conditions: (1) hypertension (≥130/85), (2) >triglycerides (≥150 mg/dL) (3) decreased HDL-C (<40 mg/dL for males and <50 mg/dL for females), (4) central obesity (≥102 cm in males or ≥88 cm in females or ≥90/≥80 for Asians), (5) hyperglycemia (≥100 mg/dL fasting). Metabolic syndrome is characterized by insulin resistance, which increases the risk of type 2 diabetes mellitus and atherosclerosis as insulin resistance causes macrophages to accumulate in walls of vessels. Patients are at increased risk of MI, coronary heart disease, and stroke.

Symptoms	Interventions
Many people have few symptoms initially but develop symptoms over time. Weight gain with central obesity. Chest pain and dyspnea. Claudication Hirsutism, acanthosis nigricans. Peripheral neuropathy. Gout.	Lifestyle changes (increased exercise, less stress, weight loss, better diet). Statin for >LDL. Fibrates, omega-C fatty acids for >triglycerides. Metformin for insulin resistance, type 2 diabetes. Antihypertensive (ARBs, ACEIs, BBs, diuretics. Assess for obstructive sleep apnea and treat as necessary. ASA prophylaxis.

DIAGNOSTIC TESTS

Metabolic syndrome tests	Normal values/Findings
Fasting glucose	<100 mg/dL. Values of 100-125 indicate prediabetes.
Hgb A1c	4-5.5%. Values of 5.7-7.4% indicate prediabetes.
Uric acid	Male: Adult>19—4-8 mg/dL or 0.24-0.47 mmol/L; Adult >60—4.2-8.2 or 0.25-0.48. Female: Adult>19—2.5-7 mg/dL or 0.15-0.41 mmol/L; Adult>60—3.5-7.3 mg/dL or 0.21-0.43 mmol/L. Increases with diabetes, hypertension, and CHF; may evidence as gout.
Lipid panel	Goals are LDL 100 mg/dL, HDL >35 mg/dL and triglycerides <150 mg/dL.
C-reactive protein (CRP) (high sensitivity immunoassay)	Indicates risk for inflammatory process, such as found with coronary artery disease. Low risk: <1 mg/dL; Average risk: 1-3 mg/dL; High risk: >10 mg/dL
Stress ECG, ultrasound/ echocardiogram	To assess risks of cardiac disease.
Polysomnography	To assess obstructive and/or central sleep apnea, commonly associated with metabolic syndrome.

HYPERTHYROIDISM

Hyperthyroidism (thyrotoxicosis) usually results from excess production of thyroid hormones (Graves' disease) from immunoglobulins providing abnormal stimulation of the thyroid gland. Other causes include thyroiditis and excess thyroid medications.

Symptoms	Interventions
Symptoms vary and may be non-specific, especially in the elderly, and include: Hyperexcitability. Tachycardia (90-160) and atrial fibrillation. Increased systolic BP, cardiac output, and myocardial consumption of O_2. Decreased SVR and diastolic BP. Poor heat tolerance, skin flushed and diaphoretic. Dry skin and pruritis (especially in the elderly). Hand tremor, progressive muscular weakness. Exophthalmos (bulging eyes). Increased appetite and intake but weight loss.	Radioactive iodine to destroy the thyroid gland. Propranolol may be used to prevent thyroid storm. Thyroid hormones are given for resultant hypothyroidism. Antithyroid medications, such as Propacil® or Tapazole® to block conversion of T4 to T3. Surgical removal of thyroid is used if patients cannot tolerate other treatments or in special circumstances, such as large goiter. Usually one-sixth of the thyroid is left in place and antithyroid medications are given before surgery.

> **Review Video: 7 Symptoms of Hyperthyroidism**
> Visit mometrix.com/academy and enter code: 923159

THYROTOXIC STORM

Thyrotoxic storm is a severe type of hyperthyroidism with sudden onset, precipitated by stress, such as injury or surgery, in those untreated or inadequately treated for hyperthyroidism. If not promptly diagnosed and treated, it is fatal. Incidence has decreased with the use of antithyroid medications but can still occur with medical emergencies or pregnancy. Diagnostic findings are similar to hyperthyroidism, and include increased T3 uptake and decreased TSH.

Symptoms	Treatment
Increase in symptoms of hyperthyroidism. Increased temperature >38.5°C. Tachycardia >130 with atrial fibrillation and heart failure. Cardiomyopathy. Hypertension. Pulmonary edema. Gastrointestinal disorders, such as nausea, vomiting, diarrhea, and abdominal discomfort. Altered mental status with delirium progressing to coma.	Controlling production of thyroid hormone through antithyroid medications, such as propylthiouracil and methimazole. Beta blockers to decrease tachycardia. Inhibiting release of thyroid hormone with iodine therapy (or lithium). Controlling peripheral activity of thyroid hormone with propranolol. Fluid and electrolyte replacement. Glucocorticoids, such as dexamethasone. Cooling blankets. Treatment of arrhythmias as needed with antiarrhythmics and anticoagulation.

HYPOTHYROIDISM

Hypothyroidism is a condition in which the thyroid does not produce adequate thyroid hormones (T3 and T4). Causes may include chronic lymphocytic (Hashimoto's) thyroiditis (an autoimmune disorder), thyroid atrophy, thyroid radiation, imbalance of iodine, drugs (lithium, iodine compounds, amiodarone, interferon-alpha, and interleukin-2), surgical removal of thyroid, and some diseases (sarcoidosis, scleroderma). A disorder of the pituitary gland (which controls hormone production of the thyroid), such as a tumor, may also cause secondary hypothyroidism.

Symptoms	Interventions
Bradycardia and reduced cardiac output and stroke volume (increasing risk of heart failure). Increased atherosclerosis. Increased SVR. Chronic fatigue. Subnormal temperature. Weight gain, hair thinning, thickened skin. Menstrual disturbance. Myxedema (rare)—mental impairment, coma.	Hormone replacement with synthetic levothyroxine (Synthroid®) based on TSH levels. (Careful monitoring of cardiac status must be done during titration as the hormone increases oxygen demand and too high a dose may result in an MI.)

TSH LEVEL

Thyroid stimulating hormone (TSH) is a hormone secreted by the pituitary gland to stimulate the release of thyroxine and triiodothyronine from the thyroid gland. Activity of the thyroid gland affects the body's metabolic rate and the function of many other body systems. The normal range for a TSH level is 2 to 7.3 micro IU/ml.

If the patient has hypothyroidism, they may also have bradycardia, decreased contractility, and a resulting decreased cardiac output. Other cardiac signs of hypothyroidism include premature ventricular contractions (PVCs) or torsades de points.

If the patient has hyperthyroidism, they may have tachycardia and be hypertensive. The patient may then complain of palpitations or dizziness. Cardiac dysrhythmias associated with hyperthyroidism include atrial fibrillation and atrial flutter.

DIAGNOSTIC THYROID TESTS

Thyroid tests	Normal values/Findings
Thyroid stimulating hormone (TSH)	0.4-4.2 microIU/mL or milliIU/L. Usually decreased with hyperthyroidism but increased with hypothyroidism.
T3 (Triiodothyronine), 20% of thyroid hormones	Free: 2.6-4.8 pg/mL or 0.04-0.07 pmol/L.
	Total adult: 70-204 ng/dL or 1.08-3.14 nmol/L
	Total >age 60: 40-181 ng/dL or 0.62-2.79 nmol/L
	Usually increased with hyperthyroidism (either T3 or T4 or both are increased) but decreased with hypothyroidism.
T4 Thyroxine (80% of thyroid hormones)	Free: 0.8-1.5 ng/dL/10-19 pmol/L.
	Total adult: 4.6-12 mcg/dL or 79-205 nmol/L
	Total >age 60: 5-10.7 mcg/dL or 86-183 nmol/L.
	Usually increased with hyperthyroidism and decreased with hypothyroidism.
Thyroid binding globulin	Increased or decreased TBG (may be a hereditary condition) can increase or decrease T4 and T3 values, resulting in misdiagnosis of hyperthyroidism or hypothyroidism, so this test can help determine if T4 and/or T3 values are indication of disease.
Thyroid binding inhibitory immunoglobulin	Increased antibodies indicated hyperthyroidism, especially that resulting from Grave's disease, an autoimmune disease that can cause symptoms of both hyperthyroidism and hypothyroidism. . Increased antibodies block action of TSH.
Iodine thyroid scan	Demonstrates "hot" spots (hyperfunctioning nodules) and "cold" spots (hypofunctioning nodules) and detects thyroiditis and thyroid dysfunction. Can differentiate hyperthyroidism from Graves' disease or Plummer's disease. Often done with radioactive iodine uptake (RAIU).
Radioactive iodine uptake (RAIU)	Can help determine if hormone levels are decreased or increased. A radioisotope is administered with the thyroid scan and the patient returns about 24 hours later so uptake can be measured to assess the amount of hormones produced in 24 hours.
Thyroid ultrasound	Can identify hypertrophy, atrophy, cysts, masses, and nodules.
Needle biopsy	Done to rule out malignancy.

Hematology

ANEMIA

Anemia may result from a number of conditions:

- Iron deficiency anemia inhibits the production of red blood cells and their ability to carry oxygen.
- Hemolytic anemia destroys red blood cells.
- Sickle cell anemia results in misshapen red blood cells with shortened survival time.
- Aplastic anemia results in decreased production of red blood cells.
- Pernicious anemia inhibits production of healthy red blood cells, resulting in misshapen cells that cannot transport oxygen.

124

Prosthetic heart valves also can cause a form of mechanical hemolysis as red blood cells may become damaged as they pass through the valves, and the red blood cells also have a shortened survival time. With all forms of anemia, cardiovascular damage can occur, especially if the condition is chronic. With most cases of mild anemia, the body is able to compensate by increasing production of red blood cells; however, over time the hemoglobin and hematocrit fall and the oxygen available to tissues decreases. The decreased oxygen supply to the heart can accentuate angina and increase fatigue and exercise intolerance. The heart has to work harder, resulting in tachycardia and left ventricular hypertrophy, which can lead to heart failure. Over 40% of patients with MI have preexisting anemia and close to 50% of those with heart failure.

DISORDERS THAT INHIBIT PLATELET PRODUCTION

Platelet inhibition can result in thrombocytopenia with excessive bruising, petechiae, blood in stool, hematuria, epistaxis, bleeding from gums, and menorrhagia. Disorders that inhibit platelet production include:

- **Genetic disorders**: Mediterranean macrothrombocytopenia, familial platelet syndrome< Paris-Trousseau syndrome, Wiskott-Aldrich syndrome, and Fanconi anemia.
- **HIV infection:** Results in decreased production, increased destruction, and increased splenic sequestration as well as decreased platelet lifespan.
- **Vitamin deficiency**: About 20% of those with megaloblastic anemia (vitamin B12 deficiency) exhibit mild thrombocytopenia. Bone marrow suppression may also result from folic acid deficiency, usually associated with alcoholism.
- **Paroxysmal nocturnal hemoglobinuria:** Platelet inhibition linked to bone marrow failure.
- **Aplastic anemia**: Results in pancytopenia, often beginning with thrombocytopenia and then progressing to other cell types.
- **Myelodysplastic syndromes**: Cytopenias (50% include thrombocytopenia) occur because of hypercellular marrow with dysplastic changes.
- **Acquired pure amegakaryocytic thrombocytopenia:** Megakaryocyte development inhibited by an autoimmune response.
- **Cyclic thrombocytopenia:** Period suppression of platelet production followed by rebound thrombocytosis.

MEDICATIONS/SUBSTANCES THAT INHIBIT PLATELET PRODUCTION

Platelet inhibition can occur with many different medications/substances:

- **Thiazide diuretics:** Suppress the production of megakaryocytes, the precursors of platelets and also increase destruction of platelets through an immune response.
- **Tolbutamide**: May cause myelosuppression with thrombocytopenia and leukopenia as well as aplastic and hemolytic anemia.
- **Interferon (Peginterferon alfa-2a, alfa-n3 and alfa-2b):** May cause mild myelosuppression resulting in thrombocytopenia, neutropenia, and granulocytopenia.
- **Alcohol**: Thrombocytopenia usually results from cirrhosis, but alcohol can also cause direct myelosuppression, especially with large consumption of ethanol over a number of days.
- **Cytotoxic chemotherapeutic agents**: Myelosuppression occurs during treatment but the hematopoietic system tends to recover fairly quickly after treatment although some patients, especially those with repeat treatment, may exhibit inhibition of platelet production for up to 5 years.
- **NSAIDS:** May cause myelosuppression in some patients.

- **Immunosuppressive drugs (such as corticosteroids, sirolimus, tacrolimus):** May cause dose-limited myelosuppression that decreases production of platelets.
- **DMARDS (such as methotrexate, infliximab, etanercept, ciclosporin):** May cause varying degrees of myelosuppression and thrombocytopenia.

ANTICOAGULANTS

Anticoagulants are used to prevent thrombo-emboli. All pose risk of bleeding:

Aspirin	Often used prophylactically to prevent clots and poses less danger of bleeding than other drugs.
Warfarin (Coumadin®)	Blocks utilization of vitamin K and decreases production of clotting factors and is used orally for those at risk of developing blood clots, such as those with mechanical heart valves, atrial fibrillation, and clotting disorders.
Heparin	The primary intravenous anticoagulant and increases the activity of antithrombin III. It is used for those with MI and those undergoing PCI or other cardiac surgery. Monitored by aPTT.
Low molecular weight heparin	These increase activity of antithrombin III. Used for unstable angina, MI, and cardiac surgery. Medications include dalteparin (Fragmin®), enoxaparin (Lovenox®), and heparin.
Direct thrombin inhibitors	Used for unstable angina, PCI, and for prophylaxis and treatment for thrombosis in heparin-induced thrombocytopenia [allergic response to heparin that causes a platelet count drop <50,000, usually to 30-50% of baseline, usually occurring 5-14 days after beginning heparin]. Medications include argatroban (Acova®), bivalirudin (Angiomax®), dabigatran (Pradaxa®), and antithrombin III (Thrombate III®).
Factor Xa Inhibitors	Block activity of clotting factor Xa to prevent clots. Medications include apixaban (Eliquis®), edoxaban (Savaysa®), fondaparinux (Arixtra®), and rivaroxaban (Xarelto®).

NURSING CONSIDERATIONS FOR ANTICOAGULANTS

Patients on **anticoagulants** must be monitored carefully for indications of bleeding, including bloody stools, tarry stools, hematuria, epistaxis, and bleeding gums as these may indicate that the patient is at risk of hemorrhage because of excessive anticoagulation:

- **Warfarin:** The prothrombin time/International Normalized Ratio (PT/INR) must be carefully monitored during administration. International normalized ratio (INR) normal value is <2 and 2.0 to 3.0 with anticoagulation. Critical value: >3 in patients receiving anticoagulation therapy.
- **Heparin (Unfractionated):** Incompatible with numerous drugs, including ampicillin, diazepam, dobutamine, morphine sulfate, and penicillin G and may interact with other drugs and herbs. Monitored with frequent aPTT.
- **Low molecular weight heparins**: Work similarly to heparin sodium but provide more predictable anticoagulant and do not require the frequent monitoring with aPTTs.

HYPERCOAGULOPATHY

Hypercoagulopathy (thrombophilia) can result from disorders in which the blood clots more easily, increasing risk of varicose veins, deep vein thrombosis, and emboli. Women who are pregnant with thrombophilia are at increased risk of death of the fetus because of spontaneous preterm abortion or stillbirth. Inherited causes include factor V Leiden (clotting factors resist deactivation), hyperhomocysteinemia, protein S deficiency (insufficient anticlotting protein),

126

increased factor VIII level, and prothrombin G20210A substitution. Acquired causes include SLE, cancer, sickle cell anemia, development of antiphospholipid antibodies, and congenital heart defects. Clots may block arteries throughout the body and may cause thoracic outlet symptoms, with blood flow to the upper extremities restricted. Patients are at increased risk for heart attack, stroke, cardiac dysrhythmias, and heart failure. Patients with hypercoagulopathy and dilated left ventricular dysfunction are at increased risk of developing intracardiac thrombi because of the stasis that occurs. Treatment for thrombophilia includes low-dose aspirin, anticoagulant therapy warfarin standard heparin, low molecular weight heparin, adequate hydration, compression stockings, exercise, and avoidance of some medications (oral contraceptives, HRT), smoking cessation, and weight control.

HEPARIN-INDUCED THROMBOCYTOPENIA

Heparin-induced thrombocytopenia (HIT) is a complication that occurs as a result of exposure to heparin. The onset of symptoms typically occurs 5 to 10 days after heparin therapy has been initiated.

There are two types of HIT. In cases of Type I HIT, exposure to heparin causes a change in the membrane of the patient's platelets, resulting in increased platelet aggregation. It is a benign condition that is treated by discontinuing heparin therapy.

In Type II HIT, the presence of heparin triggers an immune response that causes a decreased platelet count and platelet aggregation. Thus, Type II HIT results in a hypercoagulable state that increases the likelihood of thrombus formation and elevates the risk for developing thromboembolic disorders or disseminated intravascular coagulation (DIC).

DIAGNOSIS

If the patient's platelet level drops below 100,000 mm³ during heparin therapy, or if the patient develops a thromboembolic disorder during heparin therapy, heparin-induced thrombocytopenia (HIT) should be suspected.

HIT is typically diagnosed using an enzyme-linked immunosorbent assay (ELISA) test in conjunction with a functional assay such as a serotonin release assay (SRA). An ELISA test checks for antibodies to heparin platelet 4 complexes. An SRA test follows the release of serotonin after a blood sample is mixed with heparin. The presence of high levels of serotonin indicates the beginning of platelet aggregation. Positive results in both an ELISA and an SRA indicate HIT.

KEY ASSESSMENTS

A thorough head to toe assessment is vital in the diagnosis of heparin-induced thrombocytopenia. The nurse should frequently assess perfusion to the extremities in order to diagnose deep vein thrombosis or arterial occlusion. This includes monitoring skin color, temperature, capillary refill, and the strength of the peripheral pulses. The patient's respiratory status also should be closely monitored to ensure the quick diagnosis of any pulmonary embolism. Further, the patient should be closely monitored for chest pain, tachycardia or hypotension, as these may be signs of a myocardial infarction. Finally, any neurological changes should be reported, as subsequent deterioration may indicate a cerebral vascular accident related to HIT.

NURSING IMPLICATIONS

Because bedside nurses have constant contact with the patient, they play a key role in the diagnosis of heparin-induced thrombocytopenia (HIT). The patient should be closely monitored for signs of deep vein thrombosis or cerebral vascular accident during heparin therapy. In particular the patient's platelet count should be closely monitored, and the heparin should be discontinued if there is a decrease in the platelet count greater than 50% of the baseline. If a drop in the platelet count does occur, the physician should be notified so that the heparin therapy can be discontinued and an alternative anticoagulation therapy can be started.

HEPARIN-INDUCED THROMBOCYTOPENIA COMPLICATIONS

Heparin-induced thrombocytopenia (HIT) results in a hypercoagulable state in spite of exposure to heparin. The most prevalent complication of HIT is lower extremity deep vein thrombosis (DVT). In 20% of the cases, the DVT is severe enough to result in amputation of the patient's leg. Arterial occlusion (as opposed to venous occlusion) and related cerebral vascular accidents can also occur as a result of HIT, secondary to the thrombotic occlusion of an artery. Patients who have been diagnosed with HIT also have a significantly elevated risk for pulmonary embolism, adrenal or myocardial infarction, and renal or mesenteric artery thrombosis.

Neurology

STROKE

A stroke or cerebral vascular accident is a sudden alteration in blood flow to an area of the brain, resulting in damage to cerebral tissue. A stroke is characterized by an abrupt neurological deficit. The type and severity of neurological deficit depends upon the location and amount of brain tissue damaged.

Strokes are divided into two categories. The majority of strokes occur from the occlusion of an intracranial artery, causing ischemia of the brain tissue. This type of stroke is known as an ischemic stroke. The second type of stroke is known as a hemorrhagic stroke. This stroke involves a rupture in the wall of an intracranial artery, causing decreased blood flow to an area of the brain as well as increased intracranial pressure as blood exits the blood vessel and collects inside the skull. Only about 17% of all stroke cases are hemorrhagic in nature.

SIGNS AND SYMPTOMS

The most common symptom of a stroke is a severe headache, often described as the worst headache the patient has ever experienced. The patient may also complain of a sudden decrease or loss of sensation in the face or extremities. The decrease in sensation may be localized to one side of the body. Further, the patient may experience a sudden weakness on one side of the body, resulting in decreased coordination and difficulty walking or talking. They may also present with sudden confusion, or an outright loss of consciousness. Severe nausea and vomiting or new onset seizure activity may also occur.

Hemorrhagic stroke typically occurs as a result of a rupture of a brain aneurysm (i.e., a vascular wall weakness). It can also be caused by trauma or excessive anticoagulation. Ischemic stroke can occur as a result of atherosclerosis, clots from deep vein thrombosis or atrial fibrillation, or from a hypercoagulable state.

DIAGNOSIS

A stroke is typically suspected from the patient's presenting signs and symptoms, combined with a complete medical history. The diagnosis is then confirmed through formal testing. A patient presenting with significant neurological deficits is usually sent for a CT scan without contrast. A hemorrhagic stroke can readily be visualized using this type of imaging. If significant bleeding is not visualized, CT angiography can be done to visualize the intracerebral vasculature and thereby diagnose an ischemic stroke.

An MRI can also be done to diagnose a stroke, but in the absence of a complete patient history, a CT scan has historically been identified as the better of the two imaging options. However, findings of the large multi-center HEME stroke study, reported between 2003-2005, may revise the traditional approach. With proper training, multi-modal MRI imaging can be just as accurate as CT scans overall, and far more accurate in detecting acute, chronic, and micro-hemorrhaging.

TREATING A HEMORRHAGIC STROKE

There is no medication therapy to directly treat a hemorrhagic stroke. Steps should be taken to treat fever, seizures, and any cerebral edema that might occur from increased intracranial pressure. Platelets may be given intravenously to encourage platelet aggregation. If the patient was taking anticoagulation therapy, vitamin K or protamine may be prescribed to return the patient's PT (Prothrombin Time), PTT (Partial Thromboplastin Time), and INR (International Normalized Ratio – of measured clotting time to an established average) to normal levels.

In cases of a minor hemorrhagic stroke, the focus is on closely monitoring the patient's symptoms. Surgery is typically done only for patients who are showing a life-threatening increase in intracranial pressure as a result of blood accumulation within the skull. In such cases, a craniotomy can be done to relieve intracranial pressure.

TREATING AN ISCHEMIC STROKE

An ischemic stroke is treated by administering intravenous clot-dissolving agents, such as tPA. However, thrombolytic therapy is only beneficial if initiated within 3 hours of the onset of symptoms. Patients with a history of recent surgery or bleeding disorders are ineligible to receive tPA.

Following an ischemic stroke, the patient's blood pressure should be closely monitored. Their systolic blood pressure should be kept below 185 mm Hg, and their diastolic blood pressure should be kept less than 100 mm Hg. Calcium channel blockers are the medication of choice in treating hypertension related to stroke. Blood sugar and seizure activity should also be closely monitored and controlled.

PREVENTION

Because a stroke can have tremendous long-term physiological effects, primary prevention is key. By controlling risk factors, the patient can take steps to preventing a stroke. If the patient has hypertension or diabetes, keeping their blood pressure and blood sugar within normal limits will help decrease their risk for stroke. Other lifestyle changes that can prevent a stroke include exercising regularly, quitting smoking, and limiting alcohol consumption.

Patients can decrease their risk for ischemic stroke by controlling atherosclerosis. Eating a diet that is low in sodium and fat, and taking any statins as prescribed can decrease the rate of atherosclerotic buildup. Patients who are taking anticoagulants should take their medication as prescribed. They should be encouraged to regularly have their coagulation levels checked to ensure they are receiving an appropriate amount of medication.

Renal

ACUTE KIDNEY INJURY

Acute kidney injury (AKI) or acute renal failure is a decreased ability of the kidneys to effectively remove waste from the bloodstream and regulate fluid balance. AKI is characterized by an elevated serum creatinine and BUN.

AKI is classified into three subgroups, depending upon the cause of the renal failure. Prerenal failure is the most common type of AKI, and refers to any condition that decreases blood flow to the kidneys. Postrenal AKI refers to any condition that results in blockage of outflow from the kidney. Intrarenal or intrinsic failure refers to structural damage to the kidney that results in renal failure.

> **Review Video: AKI (Acute Kidney Injury)**
> Visit mometrix.com/academy and enter code: 780321

CAUSES OF RENAL FAILURE

Prerenal failure is caused by hypoperfusion to the kidney, typically as a result of hypotension. It may also occur during GI bleeding, cardiogenic shock, or diuresis. Decreased cardiac output, such as in cardiac tamponade or myocardial infarction, may lead to prerenal failure. Structural abnormalities within the renal artery, such as renal artery stenosis, or the development of an embolus in the renal artery may also cause prerenal failure.

Postrenal failure can be caused by anything that obstructs outflow from the kidneys. This can include urinary tract infections, renal calculi, pregnancy, or an abdominal tumor.

Intrarenal failure is primarily caused by a prolonged prerenal or postrenal state. Other causes include acute tubular necrosis or exposure to nephrotoxic substances.

SIGNS AND SYMPTOMS

In acute kidney injury (AKI), the patient will present with symptoms of fluid overload that results from improper fluid management. This includes jugular venous distention, crackles or wheezes in the lungs, ascites, and peripheral edema.

Palpation of the abdomen may aid in locating any obstructions causing postrenal failure, such as a tumor or an enlarged prostate gland.

The patient may also present with an abnormal blood pressure. They may have severe hypertension as a result of renovascular disease or glomerulonephritis. Conversely, the patient may be hypotensive as a result of congestive heart failure secondary to inadequate renal diuresis.

DIAGNOSIS

Acute kidney injury (AKI) is suspected if the patient's serum BUN and creatinine are elevated. However, the underlying cause of the AKI should be investigated in order to properly treat it. The first step in ascertaining the cause is to collect a complete medical history.

Laboratory studies that can assist in ascertaining the cause of AKI include a urinalysis, a 24-hour urine collection, urine electrolytes analysis, and a complete blood count.

Imaging studies can be performed to assess structural abnormalities within the kidney. A CT scan of the kidneys can be obtained to check for lesions or tumors.

TREATMENT

Dopamine can be given in low doses to dilate the renal arteries, resulting in increased renal circulation. It also reduces the workload of the kidney tubules by reducing sodium reabsorption. The typical dosage of Dopamine is 1 to 5 mg/kg/min to produce a renal response.

Although diuretics do not help in treating AKI, they do assist in preventing fluid overload. Furosemide is given orally to help maintain urinary output. The typical dosage of Furosemide is 20 to 40mg given orally, though that dosage can be increased if the patient continues to show signs of fluid overload.

HEMODIALYSIS
USING TO TREAT RENAL FAILURE

Hemodialysis is used for both short-term dialysis and long-term for patients with ESRD. A vascular access device, such as a catheter, fistula, or graft must be established for hemodialysis. With hemodialysis, blood is circulated outside of the body through a dialyzer, which filters the blood, usually for 3-5 hours 3 times weekly. **Continuous renal replacement therapy (CCRT)** circulates the blood by hydrostatic pressure through a semipermeable membrane. CCRT is used in critical care:

- **Continuous arteriovenous hemofiltration** (CAVH) circulates blood from an artery (usually the femoral) to a hemofilter using only arterial pressure and not a blood pump. The filtered blood is then returned to the patient's venous system, often with added fluids to offset those lost.
- **Continuous arteriovenous hemodialysis** (CAVHD) is similar to CAVH except that dialysate circulates on one side of the semipermeable membrane to increase clearance of urea.
- **Continuous venovenous hemofiltration** (CVVH) pumps blood through a double-lumen venous catheter to a hemofilter, which returns the blood to the patient in the same catheter. It provides continuous slow removal of fluid, is better tolerated with unstable patients, and doesn't require arterial access.
- **Continuous venovenous hemodialysis** is similar to CVVH but uses a dialysate to increase clearance of uremic toxins.

EFFECTS ON THE CARDIOVASCULAR SYSTEM

Patients with kidney failure have reduced production of erythropoietin, resulting in decreased production of RBCs and reduced available oxygen to the heart, while increased production of renin results in increased blood pressure, putting patients at risk for left ventricular heart failure, MI, or stroke. Additionally, **hemodialysis** may cause some degree of myocardial ischemia, and repeated episodes can lead to systolic dysregulation and risk of sudden cardiac death. Myocardial ischemia is associated with silent ST segment depression during treatment and post-treatment elevation of troponin T. Patients with large interdialytic weight gain may experience episodes of hypotension during dialysis (increasing myocardial ischemia) and may require increased sodium restriction and BP maintained to at least 90 mm Hg systolic during dialysis. When a patient with existing heart disease has an AV fistula created, the left to right shunting causes increased preload and decreased SVR. The heart compensates by increasing stroke volume and cardiac output, furthering LV overload and heart failure. Long-term hemodialysis may result in amyloidosis, which can cause stiffing of the myocardium, dysrhythmias, and heart failure. Some cardiac drugs, such as most ACE inhibitors and beta-blockers, are removed by hemodialysis and must be administered after treatment or other drugs substituted.

EFFECTS ON ALBUMIN AND ELECTROLYTE IMBALANCES

Patients on **hemodialysis** are at risk of electrolyte and albumin imbalance. While albumin levels may vary (the value is generally between 3.6 and 5.0 g/dL), patients on hemodialysis should maintain serum albumin levels >4.0 g/dL to ensure levels do not fall below the safety margin. Electrolytes must be carefully monitored to ensure that hemodialysis is maintaining the correct balance. Hyperphosphatemia, for which the patient may take sevelamer hydrochloride as a phosphorous-binding agent, occurs between hemodialysis treatments and causes vascular calcification, which in turn results in hypocalcemia because as phosphate levels increase in the serum, calcium levels fall. The decrease in serum calcium stimulates the parathyroid to secrete increased PTH. With kidney disease, the body does not respond normally to PTH, so calcium leaves the bones, resulting in osteomalacia, and builds up in the vessels, causing calcification and atherosclerosis, increasing risk of heart attack and heart failure. Additionally, vitamin D, which is needed for the body to properly utilize calcium, is not metabolized normally. Hyperkalemia occurs more often than hypokalemia with hemodialysis, but hypokalemia can lead to cardiac dysrhythmias and neuromuscular impairment.

CONTRAST-INDUCED NEPHROPATHY – IODINE BASED

Contrast-induced nephropathy (iodine based) is acute renal injury resulting from IV infusion of contrast media containing iodine. Symptoms are generally absent initially but serum creatinine increases greater than 25% from baseline within 24 to 48 hours and peaks in 3 to 5 days, returning to normal within 14 days. Patients may exhibit hypotension, urinary obstruction, hyperkalemia, and signs of metabolic acidosis. Urinary output may vary from normal to anuric. Those at risk include patients with preexisting renal disease with GFR <60 mL/min, age >75 years, anemia, hypertension, cirrhosis, multiple myeloma, increased uric acid, and heart failure. Those with an IABP in place are also at increased risk. Because treatment remains primarily supportive, preventive measures, such as minimizing the volume of the contrast medium and providing pre-hydration with NS (1 mL/kg/hr) for up to 24 hours prior to procedure, are important for those at risk. Additionally, some drugs (NSAIDs, diuretics, aminoglycosides) should be avoided when a patient is receiving a contrast medium. Treatment approaches include intermittent hemodialysis or hemofiltration to remove the contrast medium. N-acetyl cysteine and IV $NaHCO_3$ have been used both before and after the procedure, but study results have been inconclusive.

CONTRAST-INDUCED NEPHROPATHY – GADOLINIUM BASED

Contrast-induced nephropathy (gadolinium based) can occur early (within 48 hours) or be delayed up to 18 months or even longer in rare cases. Gadolinium is a paramagnetic metal ion that does not contain iodine. The disorder, nephrogenic systemic fibrosis/nephrogenic fibrosing dermopathy (NSF/FND), results in fibrosis of the internal organs and the skin, causing increasing stiffness of the joints and flexion contractures. The symptoms are similar to those of scleroderma. Those at risk are almost exclusively those with preexisting renal disorders. As a preventive measure, after age 60, all patients prescribed an MRI with gadolinium should have a serum creatinine (and eGFR) within 6 weeks prior to the MRI so that use of gadolinium can be avoided if necessary. Those on dialysis should have a treatment immediately following use of gadolinium. In addition to age, risk factors include history of renal disease, diabetes, hypertension, multiple myeloma, history of solid organ transplant, and history of liver disease. Although numerous treatment approaches have been attempted, such as UV phototherapy, plasmapheresis, and high dose IVIG, there is not yet a definitive treatment.

ELECTROLYTES MAGNESIUM, CHLORIDE, PHOSPHATE, AND BICARBONATE

Magnesium is a positively charged electrolyte that is necessary to maintain the functional integrity of the neuromuscular system. A normal magnesium level falls between 1.5 and 2.5 mEq/L.

Chloride is a negatively charged electrolyte found in blood and extracellular fluid. It is necessary to maintain normal fluid levels within the body. Normal chloride levels fall between 98 to 108 mmol/L.

Phosphate is a negatively charged ion that is necessary to maintain cellular structure and function. Normal phosphate levels fall between 2.5 to 4.5 mg/dL.

Bicarbonate is a negatively charged ion that helps maintain a normal pH within the blood. The normal bicarbonate range falls between 22 to 30 mmol/L.

ELECTROLYTES SODIUM, POTASSIUM, AND CALCIUM

Sodium is a positively charged ion that is located primarily in extracellular fluid. Sodium affects fluid balance, and also plays a role in the neuromuscular system. The normal sodium range is 135 to 145 mEq/L.

Potassium is a positive ion that can be found within cells. It is essential for normal cellular function, particularly in cardiac muscle. The normal potassium range is 3.5 to 5 mEq/L.

Calcium has a number of functions within the body, including bone metabolism, transmission of impulses within the nervous system, platelet aggregation, and cardiac muscle contraction. The normal total serum calcium level (bound calcium and free calcium) falls between 8.5 to 10.4 mEq/dL.

SIGNS AND SYMPTOMS OF HYPONATREMIA

Hyponatremia typically occurs as a result of excess fluid within the extracellular space, or by excessive excretion of sodium. Though hyponatremia can occur as a result of inadequate sodium intake, it is less likely than the previous causes.

Patients with hyponatremia may present with headache, malaise, nausea, and vomiting. As hyponatremia worsens, the patient may experience confusion and decreased reflexes. If hyponatremia is not corrected, the patient will lapse into a coma. In cases of hyponatremia, sodium must be replaced carefully. Rapid sodium replacement can result in hemorrhage, neurologic damage, and death.

SIGNS AND SYMPTOMS OF HYPERNATREMIA

Hypernatremia is an elevated sodium level within the blood. It is caused by inadequate fluid intake or by significant fluid loss such as in GI bleeding, burns, excessive diuresis, or diarrhea. Administration of hypertonic fluids can also cause hypernatremia. Excessive dietary intake of sodium rarely plays a role in hypernatremia.

Patients with hypernatremia may complain of severe thirst, muscle twitching, nausea, or vomiting. They may be lethargic, irritable, or have an altered mental status. Tachycardia and oliguria may result from a dehydrated state. In severe cases, seizures or coma may occur.

SIGNS AND SYMPTOMS OF HYPOKALEMIA

Hypokalemia is typically caused by a loss of potassium through gastrointestinal processes such as vomiting, diarrhea, laxative use, and suctioning. Excessive diuresis and hyperaldosteronism may also cause hypokalemia. Excessive sweating, diabetic ketoacidosis, alkalosis, and hypomagnesemia may also cause hypokalemia.

Mild hypokalemia has few symptoms, though the patient may experience some palpitations and a slightly elevated blood pressure. The patient may also experience muscle cramping, weakness, and constipation. Severe hypokalemia can result in decreased reflexes, paralysis, and respiratory depression.

ECG changes associated with hypokalemia include flattened T waves, ST segment depression, and a prolonged QT interval.

SIGNS AND SYMPTOMS OF HYPERKALEMIA

Hyperkalemia refers to an elevated serum potassium level. It can result from renal insufficiency, severe burns, myocardial infarction, or ketoacidosis. Hyperkalemia may also be caused by hypernatremia. Certain medications, such as potassium-sparing diuretics, ACE inhibitors, beta-blockers, NSAIDS, and lithium may also cause hyperkalemia as they interfere with normal urinary excretion.

Signs and symptoms of hyperkalemia include palpitations, lower extremity weakness, diarrhea, abdominal pain, nausea, and vomiting. ECG changes that might be indicative of hyperkalemia include a prolonged PR interval, widened QRS complexes, and peaked T waves. Severe complications related to hyperkalemia include cardiac dysrhythmias, coma, and death.

SIGNS AND SYMPTOMS OF HYPOCALCEMIA

Hypocalcemia is caused primarily by hyperparathyroidism or as a result of a malignancy. Hypocalcemia can also occur as a result of decreased calcium reabsorption secondary to renal failure. Hyperphosphatemia or hypomagnesemia can result in hypocalcemia. Medications such as antineoplastic agents, heparin, and glucagon can cause hypocalcemia. Alcoholism and poor nutrition can also lead to hypocalcemia.

Patients with hypocalcemia may show increased irritability, confusion, or anxiety. Neuromuscular signs of hypocalcemia include muscle spasms, numbness, facial twitching, and seizures. Patients with hypocalcemia may have decreased coagulation, as calcium is a necessary component for clotting.

On ECG, hypocalcemia can cause a prolonged QT interval. Cardiac dysrhythmias such as torsades de pointes and asystole can also occur.

SIGNS AND SYMPTOMS OF HYPERCALCEMIA

Hypercalcemia is primarily caused by hyperparathyroidism, multiple bone fractures, and metastatic cancer. Patients who take in too much calcium through their diet or through dietary supplements are also at risk for hypercalcemia. Hypercalcemia can be caused by a dietary deficiency in phosphate, and by William's syndrome.

Patients with mild hypercalcemia may experience confusion or lethargy. Muscle pain, weakness, or hypotonicity may also occur. The patient may experience frequent renal calculi, nausea, vomiting, and constipation. Severe cases of hypercalcemia may result in coma.

ECG changes associated with hypercalcemia include bradycardia and a shortened QT interval.

SIGNS AND SYMPTOMS OF HYPOMAGNESEMIA

Hypomagnesemia is most commonly caused by poor nutritional intake. Alcoholic patients are most likely to develop hypomagnesemia because of poor diet and poor intestinal absorption. Magnesium may be lost in the GI tract as a result of poor absorption after bowel surgery or chronic diarrhea. Other causes of hypomagnesemia include pancreatitis, excessive diuresis, and hypoparathyroidism.

Patients presenting with hypomagnesemia may have also experienced weight loss secondary to poor nutrition. They may complain of cramping in the lower extremities, muscle weakness, or spasm. They may have nausea or vomiting. Severe cases of hypomagnesemia may result in seizures, coma, and dysrhythmias such as ventricular fibrillation, ventricular tachycardia, supraventricular tachycardia, and torsades de pointes.

Common ECG changes associated with hypomagnesemia include a prolonged PR interval, widened QRS complexes, and flattened T waves.

SIGNS AND SYMPTOMS OF HYPERMAGNESEMIA

Hypermagnesemia is most commonly caused by poor magnesium excretion secondary to end-stage renal disease. Other causes of hypermagnesemia include Addison's disease, diabetic ketoacidosis, lithium intoxication, and hemolysis secondary to rhabdomyolysis. Patients who receive frequent magnesium supplements are also at risk.

Hypermagnesemia is characterized by lethargy, flushing, muscle weakness, nausea, and vomiting. Patients with hypermagnesemia may also experience hypocalcemia. In severe cases of hypermagnesemia, the patient will experience decreased deep tendon reflexes and an altered mental status. Cardiovascular effects of hypermagnesemia include bradycardia, a decreased respiratory rate, prolonged atrioventricular conduction, heart block, asystole, coma, and death.

SIGNS AND SYMPTOMS OF HYPOCHLOREMIA

Hypochloremia is caused by prolonged chloride loss, typically through vomiting, sweating, diarrhea, and renal dysfunction. A prolonged fever may also cause hypochloremia. Any condition that causes hyponatremia or hypokalemia may lead to hypochloremia. Certain medications, such as bicarbonate in dialysate for CRRT, laxatives, diuretics, and corticosteroids may also cause hypochloremia.

The most common symptoms of hypochloremia are nausea and vomiting, which typically only occurs in cases of severe hypochloremia. The patient may also complain of muscle twitching and cramps, increased deep tendon reflexes, and confusion. Severe cases of hypochloremia may cause hypoventilation and paralysis.

SIGNS AND SYMPTOMS OF HYPERCHLOREMIA

Hyperchloremia typically occurs in conjunction with other electrolyte imbalances such as metabolic acidosis, ketoacidosis, or hypernatremia. The most common cause of hyperchloremia is the excessive administration of intravenous hypertonic solutions. Medications such as corticosteroids, hormone replacements, and diuretics may contribute to the onset of hyperchloremia.

Mild hyperchloremia rarely produces signs or symptoms. Diabetic patients with hyperchloremia may have difficulty controlling blood sugar levels. Patients with severe hyperchloremia may complain of generalized weakness, nausea, vomiting, or excessive thirst. Care must be taken in diagnosing the condition, as signs and symptoms of accompanying metabolic disorders may overshadow the symptoms of hyperchloremia.

SIGNS AND SYMPTOMS OF HYPOPHOSPHATEMIA

The most common cause of hypophosphatemia is decreased dietary absorption, typically secondary to chronic alcoholism, chronic diarrhea, or a vitamin D deficiency. Hypophosphatemia can also be caused by increased excretion, typically as a result of hyperparathyroidism and excessive diuresis. Respiratory alkalosis, diabetic ketoacidosis, hypothyroidism and Cushing's syndrome may also cause hypophosphatemia.

Because phosphate is essential for cellular structure and function, signs and symptoms of hypophosphatemia may be seen in all body systems. The most common symptom of hypophosphatemia is muscle weakness and osteomalacia. In severe cases, patients may experience hypoventilation, decreased level of consciousness, seizures, coma, and cardiac dysrhythmias.

SIGNS AND SYMPTOMS OF HYPERPHOSPHATEMIA

The most common cause of hyperphosphatemia is decreased excretion secondary to renal failure. Diabetic ketoacidosis, hypoparathyroidism, and systemic infections may also cause elevated serum phosphate levels. Trauma, burns, rhabdomyolysis, and severe skeletal fractures may induce hyperphosphatemia. Prolonged hypocalcemia may also lead to hyperphosphatemia.

Mild cases of hyperphosphatemia have few signs and symptoms. A patient experiencing severe hyperphosphatemia may complain of tingling in the extremities, muscle cramps and twitching, and confusion. If untreated, hyperphosphatemia may cause seizures, hypotension, and cardiac arrest.

Patients with hyperphosphatemia may have a prolonged QT interval on an ECG.

CREATININE CLEARANCE TEST

A creatinine clearance test is done to test the glomerular filtration rate (GFR), which is the typical standard by which renal function is evaluated. Creatinine clearance is measured by checking the amount of creatinine that is present in a urine specimen collected over 24 hours. It is then compared to a serum creatinine level that is obtained after the 24-hour urine collection process is completed. A 24-hour creatinine clearance test combined with a serum creatinine test is considered to be a more accurate method of checking renal function than either test alone. If the patient's creatinine clearance is low after a period of 24 hours (with the blood Creatinine level then higher than normal), it indicates abnormally functioning kidneys.

Multisystem

SIGNS AND SYMPTOMS OF MULTI-ORGAN DYSFUNCTION SYNDROME

Multi-organ dysfunction syndrome is progressive deterioration and failure of 2 or more organ systems with mortality rates of 45-50% with 2 organ systems involved and up to 80-100% if there are ≥3 systems failing. MODS is a progression of SIRS with a documented infection, organ dysfunction, hypotension, and hypoperfusion. Cardiac function becomes depressed, acute respiratory distress syndrome (ARDS) may develop, and renal failure may follow acute tubular necrosis or cortical necrosis. Thrombocytopenia appears in about 30% of those affected and may result in disseminated intravascular coagulation (DIC). Liver damage and bowel necrosis may occur. Trauma patients and those with severe conditions, such as shock, burns, and sepsis, are particularly vulnerable, especially in those >65. MODS may be primary or secondary:

- **Primary** MODS relates to direct injury/disorder of the organ systems, resulting in dysfunction, such as with thermal injuries, traumatic pulmonary injuries, and invasive infections..
- **Secondary** MODS relates to dysfunction of organ systems not directly involved in injury/disorder but developing as the result of a systemic inflammatory response syndrome (SIRS) as the patient's immune and inflammatory responses become dysregulated.

NONCARDIAC CHEST PAIN

Noncardiac chest pain is pain that is similar in presentation to angina (pressure or severe pain in chest with may extend to neck, arms [especially left] and back) but is unrelated to coronary heart disease. Causes include:

- **Gastroesophageal reflux disease (GERD):** The most common cause of noncardiac pain. This pain is often relieved by drinking liquid and burping or taking antacids.
- **Bone/muscle disorders** of the chest, such as fibromyositis.

136

- **Esophageal abnormalities/disorders:** Contractions may cause painful spasms, or contractions may be missing, allowing food to build up in the esophagus rather than moving into the stomach.
- **Pleuritis:** Inflammation of the pleura may result in sharp pain, generally on one side.
- **Gall bladder disease:** Referred pain from the gall bladder may occur in the midscapular, back, or right shoulder area.
- Gastric ulcers.
- **Emotional stress, anxiety, panic attacks:** Patients often believe a panic attack is a heart attack, and fear then exacerbates the pain.

PATHOPHYSIOLOGY OF HYPOVOLEMIC SHOCK

Hypovolemic shock occurs when there is inadequate intravascular fluid.

- The loss may be **absolute** because of an internal shifting of fluid or an external loss of fluid, as occurs with massive hemorrhage, thermal injuries, severe vomiting or diarrhea, and injuries (such as ruptured spleen or dissecting arteries) that interfere with intravascular integrity.
- Hypovolemia may also be **relative** and related to vasodilation, increased capillary membrane permeability from sepsis or injuries, and decreased colloidal osmotic pressure that may occur with loss of sodium and some disorders, such as hypopituitarism and cirrhosis.

Hypovolemic shock is classified according to the degree of fluid loss:

- Class I: <750 ml or ≤15% of total circulating volume (TCV).
- Class II: 750-1500 ml or 15-30% of TCV.
- Class III: 1500-2000 ml or 30-40% of TCV.
- Class IV: >2000 ml or >40% of TCV.

TREATMENT

Hypovolemic shock occurs when the total circulating volume of fluid decreases, leading to a fall in venous return that in turn causes a decrease in ventricular filling and preload, indicated by decrease in right atrial pressure (RAP) and pulmonary artery occlusion pressure (PAOP). This results in a decrease in stroke volume and cardiac output. This in turn causes generalized arterial vasoconstriction, increasing afterload (increased systemic vascular resistance), causing decreased tissue perfusion.

Symptoms	Treatment
Anxiety. Pallor. Cool and clammy skin. Delayed capillary refill. Cyanosis. Hypotension. Increasing respirations. Weak, thready pulse.	Treatment is aimed at identifying and treating the cause of fluid loss and reestablishing an adequate intravascular volume of fluid through administration of blood, blood products, autotransfusion, colloids (such as plasma protein fraction), and/or crystalloids (such as normal saline). Oxygen may be given through intubation and ventilation if necessary. Medications may include vasopressors, such as dopamine.

OBSTRUCTIVE SHOCK

Obstructive shock occurs when the preload (diastolic filling of the RV) of the heart is obstructed because of obstruction to the great vessels of the heart (such as from pulmonary embolism), with excessive afterload because the flow of blood out of the heart is obstructed (resulting in decreased cardiac output), or with direct compression of the heart, which can occur when blood or air fills the pericardial sac with cardiac tamponade or tension pneumothorax. Other causes include aortic dissection, aortic stenosis, vena cava syndrome, systemic hypertension, and cardiac lesions. Obstructive shock is often categorized with cardiogenic shock because of similarities. Signs and symptoms of obstructive shock may vary depending on the underlying cause but typically include:

- Decrease in oxygen saturation.
- Hemodynamic instability with hypotension and tachycardia, muffled heart sounds.
- Chest pain.
- Neurological impairment (disorientation, confusion).
- Dyspnea.
- Impaired peripheral circulation (cool extremities, pallor).
- Generalized pallor and cyanosis.

Interventions depend on the cause and may include oxygen, pericardiocentesis (cardiac tamponade), needle thoracostomy or chest tube (pneumothorax), fluid resuscitation (hypotension), and anticoagulant therapy (pulmonary embolism).

DISTRIBUTIVE SHOCK

Distributive shock occurs with adequate blood volume but inadequate intravascular volume because of arterial/venous dilation that results in decreased vascular tone and hypoperfusion of internal organs. Cardiac output may be normal or blood may pool, decreasing cardiac output. Distributive shock may result from anaphylactic shock, septic shock, neurogenic shock, and drug ingestions.

Symptoms	Treatment
Hypotension (systolic <90mm Hg or <40mm Hg from normal), tachypnea, tachycardia (>90) (may be lower if patient receiving β-blockers. Skin initially warm, later hypoperfused. Hyper- or hypothermia (>38°C or <36° C). Hypoxemia. Alterations in mentation. Decreased Urinary output. Symptoms related to underlying cause.	Treating underlying cause and stabilizing hemodynamics: Septic shock or anaphylactic therapy and monitoring as indicated. Oxygen with endotracheal intubation if necessary. Rapid fluid administration at 0.25-0.5L NS or isotonic crystalloid every 5-10 minutes as needed to 2-3 L. Inotropic agents (dopamine, dobutamine, norepinephrine) if necessary.

SEPSIS

Sepsis is presence of infection either locally or systemically in which there is a generalized life-threatening inflammatory response. Sepsis includes the criteria for qSOFA in addition to the presence of infection and one or more of the following:

Criteria for SIRS include at least 2 of the following:

- Elevated temperature >38° C or depressed <36° C.
- Tachycardia >90 bpm.
- Tachypnea >20 pm or PaCO2 <32 mm Hg.
- Leukocytosis >12,000 or leukopenia <4000 or >10% bands.

Sepsis includes the criteria for SIRS in addition to the presence of infection and one or more of the following:

- Changes in mental status.
- Hypoxemia (<72 mm Hg) without pulmonary disease.
- Elevation in plasma lactate.
- Decreased urinary output <5 mL/kg/wt for ≥1 hour.

The quick sepsis-related organ failure assessment (qSOFA) score is used by some authorities to replace the SIRS criteria to determine those at risk of sepsis. Scores range from 0 to 3 with high risk when the score is 2 or 3.

Hypotension	Systolic BP ≤100 mm Hg	1
Tachypnea	≥22 bpm	1
Altered mentation	GCS <15	1

CARDIAC FUNCTION

Sepsis, an inflammatory response to infection, is usually associated with both tachycardia and hypotension, especially as the patient's condition deteriorates and septic shock occurs. General myocardial suppression occurs with sepsis, although the cause is not completely clear. While increased coronary blood flow is common, those with preexisting coronary heart disease may exhibit localized ischemia and even myocardial infarction. Cardiac output may vary with most patients having increased output but some decreased, requiring inotropic support (usually dobutamine), especially with evidence of ongoing hypoperfusion. SVR is decreased with sepsis, resulting in arterial and venous vasodilation from release of endothelial leukotrienes and prostaglandin and leading to hypotension and to increased vascular permeability. Increased tumor necrosis factor also increases vascular permeability. As a result, intravascular fluid volume decreases, extravascular fluid volume increases, and hypoperfusion of tissues worsens. Hypoperfusion of the kidneys can lead to metabolic acidosis, which impairs cardiac contractility and increases tachycardia and myocardial dysfunction.

INTERVENTIONS

Sepsis involves an inflammatory response to infection (most often bacteria but can be from any type of organism) and can affect many body systems. **Interventions to treat sepsis** require identifying the primary source of the infection as soon as possible and initiating treatment:

- Admission to ICU.
- Laboratory assessments: CBS, blood cultures, biomarkers (procalcitonin, presepsin), chest X-ray, abdominal ultrasound, CT, or MRI, ECG, cardiac enzymes, coagulation times, renal function tests, liver function tests, electrolytes, urine tests.
- Antimicrobial agents: Empiric IV antibiotics while awaiting laboratory findings. May vary according to the type of infection and the site of primary infection.
- Arterial line and pulmonary artery catheter for monitoring and central venous catheter for IV fluids and antibiotics. PreSep oximetry catheter to monitor blood oxygen levels.
- Surgical intervention as needed (such as drainage of abscess).
- Vasopressors as needed to support blood pressure if the patient is hypotensive.
- Supportive care: Oxygen and IV fluids (crystalloids and colloids).
- Hemodialysis and mechanical ventilation as needed.
- Corticosteroids.

FLUID MANAGEMENT

When assessing the need for **fluid management**, concerns include tachycardia, hypotension, and elevated CVP >8 mm Hg (normal 2-6 mm Hg). With hypotension, a mean arterial pressure (MAP) of less than 65 for even less than 5 minutes increases risk of myocardial injury, cardiac complications, renal failure, and death. Therefore, the goals of fluid management include: MAP >65, heart rate <95, cardiac index >2.01/min/m², CVP <8 mm Hg, and adequate perfusion of tissues. The CVP has often been used to assess the need for fluid, but it does not effectively assess fluid responsiveness, and only about half of patients are responsive to fluid resuscitation. Passive leg raising or volume challenge with 300 mL fluid may be utilized to assess responsiveness through such methods as echocardiogram or esophageal Doppler, which is more accurate than arterial pressures. Because the body is better able to compensate for hypovolemia than hypervolemia, fluid overload, which can lead to organ edema, must be avoided.

PALLIATIVE CARE

One goal of **palliative care** for the cardiac patient includes helping the patient and family understand the progression of the disease and assisting them in making decisions about interventions, such as CPR, IV antibiotics, and hemodialysis, which may prolong life in the event the patient's condition worsens. Another goal is to provide care to control symptoms in order to keep the patient as comfortable as possible. Common cardiovascular symptoms include pain, peripheral edema, pulmonary edema and associated dyspnea, nausea, fatigue, depression, and anxiety. The patient/family may benefit from medication, counseling, and education about the disease and methods to control symptoms. Palliative care may be provided during active treatment or may be part of hospice care, and if so the patient/family may need to make further decisions, such as when to turn off ICDs and LVADs and stop medical treatments although those that provide comfort may continue under hospice.

THERAPEUTIC HYPOTHERMIA

Therapeutic hypothermia is used to reduce ischemic tissue damage associated with cardiac arrest, ischemic stroke, traumatic brain/spinal cord injury, neurogenic fever, and related coma (3 on Glasgow scale). Hypothermia has a neuroprotective effect by making cell membranes less permeable. Hypothermia should be initiated immediately after an ischemic event if possible but some benefit remains up to 6 hours. Desflurane or meperidine is given to reduce the shivering response. Hypothermia to 33°C may be induced by cooled saline through a femoral catheter, reducing temperature 1.5 to 2° C per hour, with by an electronic control unit. Hypothermic water blankets covering ≥80% of body the body surface can also lower body temperature. In some cases, both a femoral cooling catheter and water blanket are used for rapid reduction of temperature. Rectal probes measure core temperature. Hypothermia increases risk of bleeding (decreased clotting time), infection (from catheter), and DVT. Rewarming is done slowly at 0.5 to 1° C/hr. through warmed intravenous fluids, warm humidified air, and/or warming blanket.

ILLICIT DRUGS, ALCOHOL AND NICOTINE

Illicit drugs: Heroin and morphine use increases risks of bacteremia, endocarditis and depressed cardiac function, leading to sudden cardiac arrest. Cocaine and amphetamines can suppress the sympathetic nervous system and cause cardiac ischemia, various arrhythmias (PVCs, AF, VT), myocardial infarction (despite lack of coronary artery disease), endocarditis, dilated cardiomyopathy, pneumopericardium, pneumothorax as well as acute rupture of the aorta. Hallucinogens can cause SVT and myocardial infarction. Cannabis can cause tachycardia and increased cardiac output in low does and bradycardia and hypotension in high.

Alcohol can lead to increased blood pressure and increased triglycerides because it increases catabolism of VLDL, the lipoprotein that carries triglycerides, as well as alcoholic cardiomyopathy with left ventricular dysfunction from long-term use and stress-induced (Takotsubo) cardiomyopathy from the stress of withdrawal. Excessive use of alcohol can also lead to obesity, which further stresses the cardiovascular system.

Nicotine increases atherosclerosis and causes vasoconstriction and inflammation of the vessels, resulting in increased blood pressure, tachycardia, and coronary spasms. Nicotine may also cause cardiac arrhythmias, such as AF, and lead to increased risk of heart failure, MI, stroke, aortic aneurysm, and sudden death.

CMC Practice Test

1. A 72-year-old man with chronic systolic congestive heart failure is hospitalized due to worsening of his symptoms. He is initially stable, but on the second day of his hospitalization, he suddenly develops chest pain, worsening cough, and rapidly worsening shortness of breath. An electrocardiogram reveals an acute, left-sided, ST-segment elevation myocardial infarction. What is the most likely cause of his shortness of breath?

    a. Pulmonary embolism
    b. Pneumonia
    c. Pulmonary edema
    d. Reactive airway disease

2. A 47-year-old woman presents to the hospital with a blood pressure of 220/130 mm Hg. She is confused and restless on arrival and is unable to answer questions. Her family reports that she complained of a bad headache and nausea earlier in the day. Her husband notes that she stopped taking her blood pressure medications over the past few days because she did not feel like she needed them anymore. What is the most appropriate treatment approach?

    a. Slowly lower the patient's systolic blood pressure to 120 mm Hg with intravenous (IV) antihypertensive medication, and then switch to oral antihypertensive medication for maintenance.
    b. Slowly lower the patient's diastolic blood pressure to 85 mm Hg with oral antihypertensive medication, and then adjust the dose of antihypertensive medication to maintain blood pressure.
    c. Rapidly lower the patient's systolic blood pressure to 120 mm Hg with oral antihypertensive medication, and then adjust the dose of antihypertensive medication to maintain blood pressure.
    d. Rapidly lower the patient's diastolic blood pressure to 100 mm Hg with IV antihypertensive medication, and then gradually reduce the diastolic pressure to 85 mm Hg with oral antihypertensive medication.

3. A routine x-ray shows that a patient has an asymptomatic descending thoracic aortic aneurysm. The aneurysm has a diameter of 4 cm. What is the recommended initial management?

    a. Beta-blockers for aggressive blood pressure control and surveillance
    b. Surveillance only
    c. Surgical correction
    d. Aspirin, aggressive blood pressure control with a beta-blocker, an angiotensin-converting enzyme inhibitor, and surveillance

4. A patient complains of right-sided calf pain. The nurse decides to evaluate the patient for a possible deep venous thrombosis (DVT). All of the following signs or symptoms are typical of a DVT EXCEPT

    a. unilateral swelling of the calf.
    b. warmth.
    c. skin breakdown.
    d. superficial venous dilation.

5. What is the most serious acute complication associated with coronary artery stenting?

    a. Stent fracture
    b. Stroke
    c. Myocardial infarction
    d. Renal failure

6. The nurse is caring for a 72-year-old man who was admitted to the hospital to rule out acute coronary syndrome. While the nurse is in the room talking to the patient, he suddenly clutches his chest and then falls back on his bed unresponsive. The nurse calls for help and begins cardiopulmonary resuscitation. A team arrives with the crash cart and attaches a monitor/defibrillator to the patient's chest. The monitor reveals asystole. What should the next immediate action be?

    a. Shock the patient.
    b. Resume chest compressions.
    c. Insert an advanced airway.
    d. Give 1 mg of epinephrine intravenously.

7. Major mechanical complications of acute myocardial infarction include all of the following EXCEPT

    a. rupture of the left ventricular free wall.
    b. rupture of the interventricular septum.
    c. the development of mitral regurgitation.
    d. the development of aortic regurgitation.

8. A 68-year-old woman presents with acute substernal chest pain and dyspnea. An electrocardiogram reveals deep T-wave inversion with QT-interval prolongation. Laboratory analysis reveals very mild elevation of troponin and cardiac enzymes. The patient had no history of cardiac disease. Shortly before her symptoms developed, she had been told that her daughter and grandchild had been killed in a car accident. Echocardiography showed left ventricular (LV) apical ballooning with dyskinesis of the apical one-half of the LV. Coronary angiography demonstrated only mild coronary atherosclerosis. When the patient was reevaluated weeks later, it was shown that she had recovered normal LV function. What did this patient most likely experience?

    a. Psychosomatic chest pain
    b. Stress-induced (takotsubo) cardiomyopathy
    c. A myocardial infarction
    d. Hypertrophic cardiomyopathy

9. Which of the following arterial blood gas values is abnormal?

    a. pH, 7.38
    b. PCO_2, 43 mm Hg
    c. PaO_2, 99 mm Hg
    d. HCO_3, 14 mEq/L

10. When listening to a patient's heart sounds, the nurse notes that the first heart sound is followed by a high-pitched, holosystolic murmur heard best at the apex. The murmur sounds like it is radiating to the patient's axilla. What does this murmur most likely indicate?

    a. Mitral regurgitation
    b. Mitral stenosis
    c. Aortic regurgitation
    d. Aortic stenosis

11. A contraindication for continuous positive airway pressure is when a patient has signs and symptoms of

    a. cardiogenic pulmonary edema.
    b. a pneumothorax.
    c. pneumonia.
    d. chronic obstructive pulmonary disease.

12. A 30-year-old woman complains of chest pain and palpitations and is subsequently diagnosed with pericarditis. An echocardiogram reveals signs of a pericardial effusion. Vital signs are as follows: blood pressure, 117/68 mm Hg; respiratory rate, 15 breaths/min; heart rate, 94 beats/min; temperature, 98.5°F; and oxygen saturation, 100% on room air. The patient has no significant medical history. What is the most appropriate way to proceed at this time?

    a. Schedule a pericardiocentesis to drain the pericardial fluid, and treat the underlying condition.
    b. Treat the underlying condition, but do not drain the effusion.
    c. Schedule a surgical pericardiectomy to drain the effusion, and treat the underlying condition.
    d. Monitor the patient with telemetry until the effusion resolves.

13. A faint heart murmur that can be heard only when concentrating is most likely what grade?

    a. Grade I
    b. Grade II
    c. Grade III
    d. Grade IV

14. A patient is being discharged from the hospital with a new diagnosis of atrial fibrillation. He has started warfarin for anticoagulation. What should the target range of his international normalized ratio be?

    a. 1.0–2.0
    b. 1.5–2.5
    c. 2.0–3.0
    d. 3.0–4.0

15. A 28-year-old woman is admitted to the nurse's unit with suspected endocarditis. The patient appears acutely ill, and it is decided that antibiotic therapy should be started as soon as possible. In what manner should blood cultures be obtained in this case?

a. Obtain one blood culture immediately, then start empiric antibiotic therapy; collect two more blood samples over the next 12–24 hours.

b. Start empiric antibiotic therapy immediately, and then collect three blood samples as soon as possible.

c. Obtain three blood cultures over a 1-hour period before beginning empiric antibiotic therapy.

d. Collect three blood samples over a 24-hour period before beginning empiric antibiotic therapy.

16. A patient presents with anxiety, palpitations, tremor, heat intolerance, and weight loss. Laboratory studies reveal that the patient has low thyroid-stimulating hormone and high triiodothyronine (i.e., T3) and thyroxine (i.e., T4). Which of the following medications would be useful in relieving the patient's palpitations?

a. Captopril

b. Hydralazine

c. Amlodipine

d. Propranolol

17. A nurse's patient is being discharged with warfarin as a new medication. The nurse should instruct the patient to avoid which of the following?

a. Green, leafy vegetables

b. Rivaroxaban

c. Multivitamins

d. Acetaminophen

18. An indirect or estimated value that can be obtained from pulmonary artery catheterization as opposed to a direct measurement is

a. central venous pressure.

b. pulmonary artery wedge pressure.

c. pulmonary vascular resistance.

d. right-sided intracardiac pressure.

19. A patient presents to the hospital after experiencing a sudden onset of numbness in the right side of her face and her right arm. She also has drooping of the right side of her mouth and right arm weakness. Computed tomography reveals that the patient has suffered an acute ischemic stroke. When should cardiac monitoring be used in a patient who has had an acute ischemic stroke?

a. Cardiac monitoring is recommended during the first 24 hours after ischemic stroke onset in all patients.

b. Cardiac monitoring is not necessary if the patient remains alert and responsive after the stroke.

c. Cardiac monitoring is only necessary if the electrocardiogram shows abnormalities, such as concomitant acute cardiac ischemia.

d. Cardiac monitoring is not necessary unless there is high suspicion that a cardiac complication is related to the stroke.

20. During what time period should a patient be monitored for heparin-induced thrombocytopenia after starting heparin therapy?
   a. Over the first 5–10 days after initiating therapy
   b. Over the first 3–4 weeks after initiating therapy
   c. After the patient has been on therapy for over 2 weeks
   d. After the patient has been on therapy for over 1 month

21. Which of the following medications has been shown to play a role in preventing congestive heart failure?
   a. Calcium channel blockers
   b. Angiotensin-converting enzyme inhibitors
   c. Anticoagulants
   d. Loop diuretics

22. A patient presents with palpitations, dizziness, nausea, and chest discomfort. The patient is quickly placed on a cardiac monitor, which reveals a polymorphic ventricular tachycardia that is identified as torsade de pointes. Which of the following electrolyte imbalances is a risk factor for developing torsade de pointes?
   a. Hypercalcemia
   b. Hypomagnesemia
   c. Hyperkalemia
   d. Hypochloremia

23. Permanent cardiac pacing is a beneficial option with all of the following clinical conditions EXCEPT
   a. symptomatic sinus bradycardia.
   b. torsade de pointes associated with hypokalemia.
   c. second-degree atrioventricular Mobitz II block.
   d. significant carotid sinus hypersensitivity.

24. A patient with a history of congestive heart failure presents with dyspnea, cough, and peripheral edema. On physical examination, the patient is found to be hypotensive with diminished distal pulses. Crackles in the lungs and chest x-ray findings indicate the presence of pulmonary congestion. Laboratory testing reveals that renal insufficiency is also present. What initial treatment should the nurse give the patient?
   a. Loop diuretics
   b. Thiazide diuretics
   c. Angiotensin-converting enzyme inhibitors
   d. Vasodilators

25. A patient presents to the hospital with atrial fibrillation. It is unknown how long the patient has been in atrial fibrillation. The patient did not convert to a regular sinus rhythm with medical treatment, so it is decided to continue the patient on medication for rate control and anticoagulation. It is also decided that cardioversion should be attempted. Ideally cardioversion should be attempted
   a. immediately to eradicate the arrhythmia.
   b. after the patient has had 3–5 days of anticoagulation.
   c. after the patient has had 3–4 weeks of anticoagulation.
   d. after 3–4 months of anticoagulation.

26. A patient presents with complaints of dyspnea, a feeling of chest fullness, and fatigue. On physical examination, the patient is found to have elevated jugular venous pressure, hypotension, pulsus paradoxus, and tachycardia. An electrocardiogram shows sinus tachycardia, low voltage, and beat-to-beat alterations in the QRS complexes. What is the most likely diagnosis?

    a. Acute myocardial infarction
    b. Pulmonary embolus
    c. Aortic dissection
    d. Cardiac tamponade

27. Several hours after undergoing a cardiac catheterization procedure a patient complains of severe, diffuse, abdominal pain. He then has an episode of bloody diarrhea. What does the nurse suspect may be the cause of his symptoms?

    a. Mesenteric ischemia
    b. Cholecystitis
    c. Acute renal failure
    d. Gastric ulceration

28. Cor pulmonale is a common complication of what disease state?

    a. Chronic atrial fibrillation
    b. Pulmonary hypertension
    c. Pneumonia
    d. Coronary artery disease

29. A patient is brought to the hospital after experiencing cardiac arrest. He was resuscitated in the field and then brought to the hospital for further treatment. The therapeutic (induced) hypothermia protocol is quickly instituted for the patient. The aim of therapeutic hypothermia after a cardiac arrest is to prevent

    a. neurological injury.
    b. pulmonary injury.
    c. renal failure.
    d. a stroke.

30. A 77-year-old patient complains of chest discomfort and seems confused as compared to baseline. A quick check of the vital signs reveals the following: heart rate, 44 beats/min; respiratory rate, 18 breaths/min; blood pressure, 86/49 mm Hg; and oxygen saturation, 89%. His pulse is palpable. He is placed on oxygen by nasal cannula, intravenous (IV) access is obtained, and a cardiac monitor/defibrillator is attached. What should the next step in this patient's care?

    a. Begin transcutaneous pacing.
    b. Administer dopamine, 2–10 mcg/min IV.
    c. Administer a 0.5-mg atropine bolus IV.
    d. Administer epinephrine, 2–10 mcg/min IV.

31. What life-threatening arrhythmia is associated with the long QT syndrome?

    a. Wolff-Parkinson-White syndrome
    b. Sick sinus syndrome
    c. Torsade de pointes
    d. Ventricular fibrillation

32. A 72-year-old man complains of chest pain, shortness of breath, and dizziness. His vital signs are as follows: oxygen saturation, 95%; respiratory rate, 20 breaths/min; heart rate,120 beats/min; and blood pressure, 78/50 mm Hg. His blood pressure 1 hour before this was 122/75 mm Hg. His electrocardiogram is normal other than the presence of tachycardia. What action should be taken first?

  a. Draw arterial blood gases.
  b. Begin giving the patient 100% oxygen through a nasal cannula.
  c. Give the patient a low dose of nitroglycerin while monitoring blood pressure.
  d. Establish intravenous access immediately with a large-bore intravenous catheter.

33. When should transesophageal echocardiography be the initial test of choice as opposed to transthoracic echocardiography?

  a. With suspected pericardial effusion
  b. To evaluate left ventricle ejection fraction
  c. With suspected cardiomyopathy
  d. With suspected acute aortic dissection

34. A patient presents with chest pain, severe hypotension, tachycardia, agitation, and cool, clammy skin. Lung examination reveals diffuse crackles. Other physical examination findings include diminished distal arterial pulses and increased jugular venous pressure. Which of the following combination of signs and symptoms makes cardiogenic shock a more likely diagnosis than hypovolemic or distributive shock?

  a. Diffuse crackles in the lungs and increased jugular venous pressure
  b. Chest pain and tachycardia ·
  c. Diminished distal arterial pulses and cool, clammy skin
  d. Severe hypotension and agitation

35. A 56-year-old woman is monitored in the inpatient telemetry unit. It is noted that she had an episode of non-sustained ventricular tachycardia. The patient was asymptomatic during the episode. What diagnostic test should be performed for further evaluation?

  a. Cardiac computed tomography or magnetic resonance imaging
  b. Transthoracic echocardiography
  c. Angiography
  d. Cardiac enzymes and troponin levels

36. If a patient has already received fibrinolytic therapy for an acute ST-segment elevation myocardial infarction, when is additional treatment with percutaneous coronary intervention (PCI) most likely to be recommended?

  a. If possible, all patients should receive PCI 2 hours after receiving fibrinolytic therapy.
  b. Patients who have hemodynamic instability, despite fibrinolytic therapy, should receive PCI.
  c. Stable patients who have been found to have an occluded infarct-related artery should receive PCI.
  d. If the fibrinolytic therapy was given within the past 2 hours, the patient should receive PCI.

37. **A typical presentation of a patient with unstable angina is best described as chest discomfort or pain that is**
   a. difficult to describe, begins at rest, and lasts for longer than 20 minutes.
   b. described as sharp and stabbing and improves when the patient is sitting up or leaning forward.
   c. difficult to describe, begins while the patient is exercising, and resolves within 2–5 minutes after resting.
   d. described as sharp and is reproducible on examination.

38. **A patient being monitored on telemetry suddenly develops a completely erratic rhythm on the monitor with no distinguishable waves. When the nurse comes into the room, the patient is unarousable. What dysrhythmia is likely to be the cause?**
   a. Atrial flutter
   b. Atrial fibrillation
   c. Ventricular flutter
   d. Ventricular fibrillation

39. **Binge drinking puts patients at significantly higher risk for which cardiac dysrhythmia?**
   a. Atrial fibrillation
   b. Ventricular fibrillation
   c. Bradycardia
   d. Premature ventricular contractions

40. **A 34-year-old man is brought to the emergency department because of chest pain. It is quickly determined that he is experiencing an acute ST-segment elevation myocardial infarction as a result of cocaine ingestion. How should this patient's initial treatment differ from other instances of acute coronary syndrome?**
   a. Aspirin use should be avoided in the acute setting.
   b. Beta-blocker use should be avoided in the acute setting.
   c. Supplemental oxygen use is not necessary in the acute setting.
   d. Nitroglycerin use should be avoided in the acute setting.

41. **What is the recommended length of time between initial medical contact and primary percutaneous coronary intervention in a patient with an ST-segment elevation myocardial infarction ("door-to-balloon" time)?**
   a. 30 minutes
   b. 90 minutes
   c. 2 hours
   d. 4 hours

42. **A patient presents with chest pain, elevated jugular venous pressure, cyanosis, a right ventricular heave, and sinus tachycardia on electrocardiogram. He has been bedridden for the past week following surgery. Vital signs are as follows: blood pressure, 100/60 mm Hg; respiratory rate, 40 breaths/min; heart rate, 115 beats/min; and oxygen saturation, 80% on room air. The patient remains persistently hypotensive. What should be done first?**
   a. Ventilation/perfusion scan
   b. Computed tomography pulmonary angiogram
   c. Administration of streptokinase
   d. Administration of warfarin

43. A nurse is caring for a patient with acute respiratory distress syndrome who is intubated in the intensive care unit. The patient is being kept sedated with benzodiazepines at this time. In addition to improving tolerance of mechanical ventilation, sedation is specifically useful in this patient for which of the following reasons?

    a. It will improve blood flow.
    b. It acts as an analgesic.
    c. It decreases glucose consumption.
    d. It decreases oxygen consumption.

44. A 19-year-old patient presents with the sudden onset of chest pain and dyspnea. His vital signs are as follows: respiratory rate, 30 breaths/min; blood pressure, 100/60 mm Hg; heart rate, 110 beats/min; and oxygen saturation, 88%. Physical examination reveals diminished breath sounds on the left side. Chest radiograph reveals a hyperlucent line along the left chest wall. All of the following are risk factors associated with this patient's condition EXCEPT

    a. hypertension.
    b. gender.
    c. mechanical ventilation.
    d. smoking.

45. A patient presents with cardiogenic shock following an acute myocardial infarction (MI). How should this patient's treatment differ from that of acute MI without shock?

    a. Lidocaine should be used in higher doses than usual.
    b. Calcium channel blockers should be avoided.
    c. Clopidogrel should be given before angiography.
    d. Aspirin therapy should be avoided.

46. Which of the following is the most specific and sensitive cardiac blood marker for acute myocardial infarction?

    a. Troponin
    b. Creatine kinase–myoglobin
    c. Total creatine kinase
    d. B-type natriuretic peptide

47. ST-segment elevation that is seen diffusely in most or all limb and precordial leads is most likely indicative of

    a. acute myocardial infarction.
    b. cardiac tamponade.
    c. pericarditis.
    d. left ventricular hypertrophy.

48. An electrocardiogram (ECG) performed on a patient on the telemetry floor reveals variable PR intervals, a fast atrial rate, and a slow ventricular rate. The atrial beats and ventricular beats do not appear to be related. This patient is likely to have which type of atrioventricular (AV) block listed below?

    a. First-degree AV block
    b. Second-degree AV Mobitz I block
    c. Second-degree AV Mobitz II block
    d. Third-degree AV block

49. An 81-year-old woman is on her third day of hospitalization for an exacerbation of her chronic congestive heart failure. Her symptoms have improved over the course of her stay. The nurse notes that her vital signs are as follows: oxygen saturation (SaO_2), 81% on room air; respiratory rate, 18 breaths/min; heart rate, 90 beats/min; and blood pressure, 131/88 mm Hg. Her SaO_2 on room air for the past day has been over 95%. She appears to be breathing comfortably at this time and does not appear ill. What is the first thing that the nurse should do?

   a. Place the patient on 100% oxygen by nasal cannula.
   b. Place the patient on 100% oxygen by non-rebreather mask.
   c. Recheck the patient's pulse oximetry.
   d. Page the patient's physician immediately.

50. Which of the following patients would be eligible for an exercise electrocardiogram stress test?

   a. An active 65-year-old woman with a right bundle branch block
   b. An active 68-year-old woman who has a paced ventricular rhythm
   c. An active 62-year-old man with a left bundle branch block
   d. An active 60-year-old man with Wolff-Parkinson-White syndrome

Answer Key and Explanations

1. C: The medical history of the patient described in the question is key to discovering the most likely cause of his shortness of breath. He already had a history of congestive heart failure, which likely developed into acute decompensated heart failure (ADHF) due to his ST-segment elevation myocardial infarction. The ADHF is a fairly common cause of acute respiratory distress and is associated with the rapid accumulation of fluid in the lungs (pulmonary edema). Although a pulmonary embolism, pneumonia, and reactive airway disease may all cause dyspnea, cough, and chest pain, they are less likely in this case due to the patient's history.

2. D: The patient described in the question is experiencing a hypertensive emergency with associated hypertensive encephalopathy. In this situation, a patient's diastolic blood pressure should be rapidly lowered to around 100 mm Hg with intravenous antihypertensive medication (with the maximum initial decrease 25% or less of the presenting value). This initial decrease in blood pressure should take place over 2–6 hours. Once the blood pressure is controlled, the patient should be switched to oral therapy, and the diastolic blood pressure should gradually be reduced to about 85 mm Hg over the next 2–3 months. While the severity of the symptoms calls for rapid lowering of the blood pressure, if the blood pressure is lowered too much over a short period of time, other complications, such as renal failure, could occur.

3. A: In an asymptomatic patient with a descending thoracic aortic aneurysm with a diameter of less than 6 cm, medical management is recommended. This includes aggressive blood pressure control with beta-blockers as part of the regimen, surveillance for signs and symptoms, and serial imaging to evaluate growth and structure. Surgery is indicated if the patient is symptomatic, if the descending aortic aneurysm is 6–7 cm or greater, if the aneurysm has an accelerated growth rate, or if there is evidence of dissection.

4. C: There are no physical examination findings that can definitively diagnose a deep venous thrombosis (DVT), but certain findings may help guide further action. Findings that may be associated with a DVT include a palpable cord, calf or thigh pain, unilateral edema, warmth, tenderness, erythema, and superficial venous dilation. Skin breakdown is not a typical sign of DVT.

5. B: Stroke is the most serious acute complication associated with coronary artery stenting in patients with carotid stenosis. Stroke may result from thromboembolism, hypoperfusion, intracerebral hemorrhage, or cerebral hyperperfusion. Stent fractures, myocardial infarctions, and renal dysfunction are other complications of coronary artery stenting, but stroke is considered the most serious.

6. B: Asystole is not a rhythm that can be shocked into regularity. One of the most important parts of advanced cardiac life support is to minimize interruptions in chest compressions. A team member should ensure that the patient has good intravenous access; 1 mg of epinephrine can be given every 3–5 minutes, but chest compressions should continue while this is taking place. The patient may need to have an advanced airway placed, but once again, chest compressions should be continued while preparations are made.

7. D: The three major medical complications of acute myocardial infarction include rupture of the left ventricular free wall, rupture of the interventricular septum, and the development of mitral regurgitation (often due to papillary muscle rupture). If a new murmur develops, if there is evidence of hypoperfusion, or if severe decompensated heart failure occurs, suspicion of a mechanical complication is warranted. The diagnosis is often made with echocardiography. Each of these complications can lead to cardiogenic shock and death if not treated emergently.

8. B: Stress-induced (takotsubo) cardiomyopathy is characterized by transient systolic dysfunction of the apical segment of the left ventricle (LV), LV apical ballooning, electrocardiographic changes, mild elevation of troponin and cardiac enzymes, and absence of obstructive coronary artery disease. Symptoms may be similar to a myocardial infarction, but the fact that there is only very mild elevation in troponin and the patient's quick recovery should make you think about other options. The combination of characteristic findings described here and the preceding stressor indicate stress-induced cardiomyopathy. It is frequently triggered by an acute medical illness or an intense emotional or physical stress.

9. D: The range of normal arterial blood gas values varies slightly between laboratories, but the normal ranges are as follows: pH, 7.36–7.44; PCO_2, 36–44 mm Hg; PaO_2, more than 80 mm Hg (if new values are substantially different from old values then they may be considered abnormal even if more than 80 mm Hg); and HCO_3, 21–27 mEq/L.

10. A: The murmur of mitral regurgitation may vary, but in its typical presentation, it is holosystolic, begins immediately after S1, is heard best over the apex, and may radiate to the axilla or back. Mitral valve stenosis has a rumbling, mid-diastolic murmur and is heard best with the bell of the stethoscope over the left ventricular impulse. Aortic regurgitation is heard as a blowing, early diastolic murmur that radiates toward the cardiac apex and is often heard best along the left sternal border. Aortic valve stenosis causes a mid-systolic murmur that is typically loudest in the right second intercostal space and may radiate to the carotids.

11. B: Continuous positive airway pressure (CPAP) is contraindicated in patients who are suspected of having a pneumothorax, because the CPAP would likely cause an increased buildup of air (and therefore tension) in the chest cavity, which may result in further deterioration of the patient's condition. CPAP has been shown to be helpful as noninvasive positive pressure ventilation in other causes of acute respiratory failure, such as cardiogenic pulmonary edema, pneumonia, and chronic obstructive pulmonary disease.

12. B: If a patient with a pericardial effusion is hemodynamically stable and has no evidence of cardiac tamponade, immediate drainage of the effusion is not required. The underlying cause of the effusion should be determined and appropriate medical treatment instituted. If it is determined that the patient is stable, she can be treated as an outpatient. She should be educated about symptoms of increasing pericardial effusion, and outpatient follow-up should be scheduled.

13. A: Grade I heart murmurs are very faint, but with practice, they can be heard when concentrating. Grade II murmurs are still faint but are more easily heard. Grade III murmurs are moderately loud and not associated with a thrill. Grade IV murmurs are loud and may be associated with a thrill. Grade V murmurs are very loud and associated with a thrill. Grade VI murmurs are very loud, can be heard even without a stethoscope on the chest, and are associated with a thrill.

14. C: An international normalized ratio between 2.0 and 3.0 is recommended for most patients with atrial fibrillation to prevent embolization of atrial thrombi. If the patient has other risk factors, his target range may need to be adjusted.

15. C: It is very important to obtain blood samples before antibiotic therapy to increase the likelihood of identifying the infecting organism. In patients who are acutely ill, three separate blood cultures should be obtained over a 1-hour period, and then empiric antibiotic therapy should be started. Once the organism is identified, the patient can be switched over to more specific antimicrobial agents. If the illness is subacute and the patient is not critically ill, three blood cultures should still be obtained before antibiotic therapy, but they can be collected over a longer period of time. In these subacute cases, it may be preferable to delay therapy for 1–3 days until the results of the blood cultures are back.

16. D: Beta-blockers, such as propranolol and atenolol, are useful in relieving palpitations and slowing the heart rate in patients with hyperthyroidism. Beta-blockers, however, do not treat the underlying cause of these symptoms.

17. B: Rivaroxaban is an anticoagulant that can greatly increase bleeding risk if taken concurrently with warfarin. Green, leafy vegetables and multivitamins contain vitamin K, which will decrease the effectiveness of warfarin; however, warfarin dosing can be adjusted accordingly. Patients should be educated about the importance of being consistent with their vitamin K intake so as not to alter their drug effectiveness. Acetaminophen can be taken safely with warfarin.

18. C: Pulmonary vascular resistance, systemic vascular resistance, and cardiac output can all be *estimated* from measurements obtained from pulmonary artery catheterization. Pulmonary artery catheters can *directly* measure central venous pressure, right-sided intracardiac pressure, pulmonary arterial pressure, and pulmonary artery wedge pressure.

19. A: Cardiac monitoring is recommended for all patients during the first 24 hours after the initial onset of an ischemic stroke. Cardiac monitoring is used to detect atrial fibrillation or other cardiac arrhythmias that may need to be addressed. Atrial fibrillation may suggest cardiac emboli as a possible causes of the stroke. Even if a patient is alert, does not have acute electrocardiographic abnormalities, and does not have a history of cardiac disease, it is important to monitor for cardiac arrhythmias after a stroke.

20. A: Most cases of heparin-induced thrombocytopenia occur within 5–10 days of initiating heparin therapy. It is unusual to see onset after 2 weeks.

21. B: Angiotensin-converting enzyme (ACE) inhibitors not only help control blood pressure by causing vasodilation, but they also provide extra cardiac protection beyond that of other antihypertensive medications. The reduction in vascular tone leads to improved emptying of the left ventricle. The ACE inhibitors have also been shown to attenuate the remodeling process of the ventricles that is associated with congestive heart failure.

22. B: Risk factors for developing torsade de pointes include certain electrolyte disturbances, especially hypomagnesemia and hypokalemia. Less often hypocalcemia is found to be a cause. A first-line therapy for the treatment of torsade de pointes is intravenous magnesium sulfate. It is effective for both the treatment and prevention of the long QT-related arrhythmia. These treatments have been shown to be beneficial even in patients with normal baseline serum magnesium concentrations.

23. B: Torsade de pointes associated with hypokalemia is likely reversible once the electrolyte imbalances are corrected. Permanent pacing is considered definitely beneficial and effective in patients with symptomatic sinus bradycardia, second-degree atrioventricular Mobitz II block (especially if symptomatic), or significant carotid sinus hypersensitivity.

24. D: The patient described in the question has inadequate perfusion along with signs and symptoms of volume overload. Cardiac output should be improved first, before excess volume is removed. Cardiac output can be increased by using intravenous vasodilators, inotropes, or both.

After cardiac output is improved, diuretics can be used to address volume overload. Angiotensin-converting enzyme inhibitors will not address the patient's acute symptoms.

25. C: In some patients with persistent atrial fibrillation, cardioversion to sinus rhythm is a treatment option. It is recommended that a patient be anticoagulated for 3–4 weeks before and after cardioversion to reduce the risk of thromboembolism. If it is decided that cardioversion should be done sooner, before therapeutic anticoagulation is achieved, then a transesophageal echocardiogram should be done before cardioversion to exclude the presence of an existing intracardiac thrombus.

26. D: Characteristic symptoms of cardiac tamponade include sinus tachycardia, hypotension, elevated jugular venous pressure (JVP), and pulsus paradoxus. Beat-to-beat alterations in the QRS complex seen on electrocardiogram (ECG), otherwise known as electrical alternans, are a relatively specific finding for cardiac tamponade. Hypotension and elevated JVP can be seen in cases of acute myocardial infarction (MI) and large pulmonary emboli; however, these disorders are not associated with pulsus paradoxus. In addition, acute MI is associated with characteristic ECG changes of infarction. Although aortic dissection may lead to the development of cardiac tamponade, aortic dissection in the absence of cardiac tamponade should not cause an increase in JVP.

27. A: The patient described in the question has experienced occlusion of his mesenteric artery with resultant intestinal ischemia. This complication is caused by trauma to a blood vessel or by dislodging an atherosclerotic plaque in the vessel. Systemic embolization caused by cardiac catheterization can cause cutaneous, renal, retinal, cerebral, or gastrointestinal emboli, which may or may not be clinically significant. Although renal dysfunction may be caused by a renal embolus, the bloody diarrhea and sudden onset of diffuse abdominal pain in this case make it more likely that mesenteric ischemia is the cause. Cholecystitis and gastric ulceration are not complications related to cardiac catheterization.

28. B: Cor pulmonale refers to the altered structure and function of the right ventricle of the heart. This dysfunction can result from any cause of pulmonary hypertension. Typically, cor pulmonale is slowly progressive, but in some cases, it can be acute. Symptoms include dyspnea on exertion, fatigue, exertional angina, and syncope.

29. A: One of the main purposes of therapeutic (induced) hypothermia after a resuscitated cardiac arrest is to improve neurological outcomes. Neurologic injury is the most common cause of death in patients who experience a cardiac arrest while not in the hospital.

30. C: When a patient has a bradyarrhythmia with a pulse, it is important to determine whether the bradyarrhythmia is causing hypotension, acutely altered mental status, signs of shock, ischemic chest discomfort, or acute heart failure. If none of these signs or symptoms is present, the patient can be monitored and observed. If one or more of these sign or symptoms is present, a 0.5-mg bolus of intravenous atropine should be given every 3–5 minutes (to a maximum of 3 mg). If atropine is ineffective, transcutaneous pacing, a dopamine infusion, or an epinephrine infusion should be considered.

31. C: Torsade de pointes is a distinctive form of polymorphic ventricular tachycardia in which there is a gradual change in the amplitude and twisting of the QRS complexes around the isoelectric line. It is associated with a congenital or acquired prolonged QT interval.

32. D: The acute change in blood pressure of the patient described in the question should be addressed immediately by establishing intravenous access with a large-bore intravenous catheter for the administration of fluids. As long as there is no evidence of pulmonary edema, a normal saline bolus should be given, and the patient should have a work-up for possible causes of the acute hypotension. The normal oxygen saturation is reassuring but should continue to be monitored. An arterial blood gas should be drawn, but establishing intravenous access is a priority. Nitroglycerin could worsen the patient's acute hypotension.

33. D: Transesophageal echocardiography (TEE) should be the initial test of choice in certain life-threatening situations or in cases where transthoracic echocardiography (TTE) is likely to be non-diagnostic. Examples where TEE should be the initial test include: suspected acute aortic pathology, suspected prosthetic valve dysfunction, suspected complications of endocarditis, and evaluation for thrombi in the left atrium. There are many more cases where TEE may be helpful, but often TTE is done first since it is a safer and less complicated test.

34. A: Cardiogenic shock is caused by cardiac pump failure, leading to decreased cardiac output and the inability to maintain perfusion to the vital organs. Decreased cardiac output can result in pulmonary congestion and pulmonary edema, resulting in crackles in the lungs. In hypovolemic and distributive shock there is more likely to be decreased jugular venous pressure (JVP), while in cardiogenic shock, increased JVP is often present.

35. B: Asymptomatic non-sustained ventricular tachycardia is often benign, but it is important to rule out any associated structural heart disease. In asymptomatic patients, the initial evaluation should include a thorough history and physical examination, a 12-lead electrocardiogram, transthoracic echocardiography, and exercise stress testing.

36. B: The preferred reperfusion therapy for patients with an acute ST-segment elevation myocardial infarction is percutaneous coronary intervention (PCI). Fibrinolytic therapy is usually reserved for patients who cannot receive PCI in a timely fashion. If a patient has hemodynamic instability or cardiogenic shock, PCI is the treatment of choice, even if the patient has already received fibrinolytic therapy. Not all patients will need PCI after fibrinolytic therapy. If PCI is deemed necessary, it should not be performed within the first 2 hours after the administration of fibrinolytic therapy if possible. For stable patients who are subsequently found to have an occluded infarct-related artery, it is not recommended that PCI be performed if they do not show evidence of spontaneous or significant provocable ischemia.

37. A: Unstable angina is one presentation of acute coronary syndrome. It is often reported as chest discomfort that is difficult to describe but may feel like tightness, squeezing, pressure, or aching in the chest. There may be radiation of the pain to the shoulder, arm, jaw, and neck as well as shortness of breath and sweating. Unstable angina may occur at rest without any instigation (e.g., while sleeping) and may last longer than 20 minutes. Answer B describes a typical presentation of chest pain due to pericarditis. Answer C describes a typical presentation of stable angina. Answer D describes a possible presentation of costochondritis.

38. D: Ventricular fibrillation is caused by rapid discharges from many irritable ventricular automaticity foci. This produces an irregular, rapid twitching of the ventricles, resulting in an erratic electrocardiographic (ECG) tracing with no distinguishable waves. Atrial flutter is characterized by a series of identical, rapid "flutter" waves (often described as a "saw tooth" pattern) with distinguishable, but possibly irregular QRS complexes. Atrial fibrillation often appears as a wavy baseline without distinguishable P waves and an irregular QRS response. Ventricular flutter appears as a rapid series of smooth sine waves of similar amplitude on ECG.

39. A: Atrial fibrillation has been shown to occur in up to 60% of binge drinkers, even if they did not have underlying alcoholic cardiomyopathy. Regular heavy alcohol consumption is also associated with an increase in the occurrence of atrial fibrillation.

40. B: In a patient with cocaine-associated acute myocardial ischemia or infarction, beta-blockers should not be used until the cocaine is eliminated from the body due to the risk of unopposed alpha-adrenergic stimulation. Unopposed alpha-adrenergic stimulation could lead to coronary artery vasoconstriction and systemic hypertension, causing worsening of the patient's condition. Aspirin, nitroglycerin, and oxygen remain safe and effective medications in cocaine-associated acute coronary syndrome cases.

41. B: The American College of Cardiology/American Heart Association guidelines recommend that primary percutaneous coronary intervention (PCI) be implemented within 90 minutes of first medical contact in patients with ST-segment elevation myocardial infarctions who are otherwise eligible for the procedure. Studies have shown enhanced survival with PCI as compared to fibrinolysis.

42. C: The patient described in the question most likely has a massive pulmonary embolus. Since the patient has persistent hypotension, thrombolytic therapy should be considered immediately with the aim of dissolving the embolism. Another immediate and potentially life-saving treatment option would be pulmonary arteriotomy with embolectomy. If the patient is hemodynamically stable and has no contraindications, therapy with heparin or low-molecular-weight heparin should be started for fast anticoagulation. Oral warfarin should be started on day 1, but this medication will generally take several days to achieve appropriate anticoagulation. A ventilation/perfusion scan or computed tomography pulmonary angiogram can be performed after the patient is stable to confirm the diagnosis of pulmonary embolism.

43. D: Acute respiratory distress syndrome (ARDS) is a type of hypoxemic respiratory failure caused by acute, diffuse, inflammatory lung injury in both lungs. An important part of the care for patients with ARDS involves management of hypoxemia. This is done by using high fractions of inspired oxygen, decreasing oxygen consumption, improving oxygen delivery, and careful use of mechanical ventilatory support. In this case, sedating the patient will help to relieve anxiety and agitation and maximize rest, therefore, lowering oxygen consumption. Benzodiazepines do not act as analgesics.

44. A: Hypertension itself is not a risk factor associated with pneumothoraces. Men are more likely than women to develop pneumothoraces. Mechanical ventilation can cause an imbalance of air pressure in the chest, resulting in a pneumothorax. Smoking can damage lung tissue, and damaged lung tissue is more likely to collapse. Many underlying lung diseases or chest injuries may lead to pneumothoraces.

45. B: Differences in treating patients with acute myocardial infarction complicated by cardiogenic shock as compared to treating patients without shock include holding clopidogrel until after angiography, using lidocaine in low doses, and avoiding drugs with negative inotropic properties, such as beta-blockers and calcium channel blockers, while the patient is in shock. The patient can still be treated with aspirin.

46. A: Troponin is the preferred cardiac marker for diagnosing acute myocardial infarction (MI) because it has increased sensitivity and specificity as compared with creatine kinase–myoglobin (CK-MB) and total creatine kinase (CK). Troponin is more consistently elevated in acute MIs than CK-MB. Also, CK is found in many body tissues, and can, therefore, be elevated for various reasons.

CK-MB is more specific for cardiac muscle than total CK, but it is also found in skeletal muscle, making it a less specific marker than troponin. Troponin also has enhanced prognostic value as compared to CK. B-type natriuretic peptide is a hormone used for evaluation of heart failure, not acute MI.

47. C: In pericarditis, there is J-point elevation and ST-segment elevation, which has a concave morphology that is usually diffusely seen in all leads. ST-segment elevation associated with acute myocardial infarction typically shows up in the leads corresponding to the area of infarction, rather than diffusely. The electrocardiogram in cardiac tamponade typically shows sinus tachycardia and low voltage. With left ventricular hypertrophy, ST–T-wave abnormalities are most often seen in anterolateral leads and typically consist of a horizontal or down sloping ST-segment and T-wave inversions.

48. D: A first-degree atrioventricular (AV) block is defined as a prolonged PR interval (> 0.20 seconds), resulting in slowed AV conduction. A second-degree AV Mobitz I block is the result of an intermittent block of the impulse within the AV node. The electrocardiogram shows progressive lengthening of the PR interval so that a normally occurring P wave is not followed by a QRS complex, and then the cycle begins again. A second-degree AV Mobitz II block is characterized by unpredictable failure of AV conduction. There is no change in the PR interval before or after the non-conducted P wave. A third-degree AV block occurs when there is complete failure of the AV node to conduct any impulses from the atria to the ventricles. This results in a disconnect between the atrial rhythm and the ventricular rhythm.

49. C: Since the patient appears well and is breathing comfortably, her pulse oximetry should be rechecked (possibly with a different pulse oximeter) before further action is taken. The nurse should always consider the patient's physical state instead of just relying on test values. If the patient's oxygen saturation is actually low, then she can be started on oxygen, and her physician can be contacted about the change.

50. A: Patients excluded from exercise electrocardiogram (ECG) include those who are unable to exercise sufficiently (to 85% of their predicted maximal heart rate) or those who have ECG abnormalities at rest that would interfere with test interpretation. The ECG abnormalities that exclude exercise ECG testing include the Wolff-Parkinson-White syndrome, a paced ventricular rhythm, complete left bundle branch block, more than 1 mm of ST depression at rest, ECG criteria for left ventricular hypertrophy, and patients taking digoxin. Patients who have a right bundle branch block are still candidates for diagnostic exercise ECG.

How to Overcome Test Anxiety

Just the thought of taking a test is enough to make most people a little nervous. A test is an important event that can have a long-term impact on your future, so it's important to take it seriously and it's natural to feel anxious about performing well. But just because anxiety is normal, that doesn't mean that it's helpful in test taking, or that you should simply accept it as part of your life. Anxiety can have a variety of effects. These effects can be mild, like making you feel slightly nervous, or severe, like blocking your ability to focus or remember even a simple detail.

If you experience test anxiety—whether severe or mild—it's important to know how to beat it. To discover this, first you need to understand what causes test anxiety.

Causes of Test Anxiety

While we often think of anxiety as an uncontrollable emotional state, it can actually be caused by simple, practical things. One of the most common causes of test anxiety is that a person does not feel adequately prepared for their test. This feeling can be the result of many different issues such as poor study habits or lack of organization, but the most common culprit is time management. Starting to study too late, failing to organize your study time to cover all of the material, or being distracted while you study will mean that you're not well prepared for the test. This may lead to cramming the night before, which will cause you to be physically and mentally exhausted for the test. Poor time management also contributes to feelings of stress, fear, and hopelessness as you realize you are not well prepared but don't know what to do about it.

Other times, test anxiety is not related to your preparation for the test but comes from unresolved fear. This may be a past failure on a test, or poor performance on tests in general. It may come from comparing yourself to others who seem to be performing better or from the stress of living up to expectations. Anxiety may be driven by fears of the future—how failure on this test would affect your educational and career goals. These fears are often completely irrational, but they can still negatively impact your test performance.

> **Review Video: <u>3 Reasons You Have Test Anxiety</u>**
> Visit mometrix.com/academy and enter code: 428468

159

Elements of Test Anxiety

As mentioned earlier, test anxiety is considered to be an emotional state, but it has physical and mental components as well. Sometimes you may not even realize that you are suffering from test anxiety until you notice the physical symptoms. These can include trembling hands, rapid heartbeat, sweating, nausea, and tense muscles. Extreme anxiety may lead to fainting or vomiting. Obviously, any of these symptoms can have a negative impact on testing. It is important to recognize them as soon as they begin to occur so that you can address the problem before it damages your performance.

Review Video: 3 Ways to Tell You Have Test Anxiety
Visit mometrix.com/academy and enter code: 927847

The mental components of test anxiety include trouble focusing and inability to remember learned information. During a test, your mind is on high alert, which can help you recall information and stay focused for an extended period of time. However, anxiety interferes with your mind's natural processes, causing you to blank out, even on the questions you know well. The strain of testing during anxiety makes it difficult to stay focused, especially on a test that may take several hours. Extreme anxiety can take a huge mental toll, making it difficult not only to recall test information but even to understand the test questions or pull your thoughts together.

Review Video: How Test Anxiety Affects Memory
Visit mometrix.com/academy and enter code: 609003

Effects of Test Anxiety

Test anxiety is like a disease—if left untreated, it will get progressively worse. Anxiety leads to poor performance, and this reinforces the feelings of fear and failure, which in turn lead to poor performances on subsequent tests. It can grow from a mild nervousness to a crippling condition. If allowed to progress, test anxiety can have a big impact on your schooling, and consequently on your future.

Test anxiety can spread to other parts of your life. Anxiety on tests can become anxiety in any stressful situation, and blanking on a test can turn into panicking in a job situation. But fortunately, you don't have to let anxiety rule your testing and determine your grades. There are a number of relatively simple steps you can take to move past anxiety and function normally on a test and in the rest of life.

Review Video: How Test Anxiety Impacts Your Grades
Visit mometrix.com/academy and enter code: 939819

Physical Steps for Beating Test Anxiety

While test anxiety is a serious problem, the good news is that it can be overcome. It doesn't have to control your ability to think and remember information. While it may take time, you can begin taking steps today to beat anxiety.

Just as your first hint that you may be struggling with anxiety comes from the physical symptoms, the first step to treating it is also physical. Rest is crucial for having a clear, strong mind. If you are tired, it is much easier to give in to anxiety. But if you establish good sleep habits, your body and mind will be ready to perform optimally, without the strain of exhaustion. Additionally, sleeping well helps you to retain information better, so you're more likely to recall the answers when you see the test questions.

Getting good sleep means more than going to bed on time. It's important to allow your brain time to relax. Take study breaks from time to time so it doesn't get overworked, and don't study right before bed. Take time to rest your mind before trying to rest your body, or you may find it difficult to fall asleep.

> **Review Video: The Importance of Sleep for Your Brain**
> Visit mometrix.com/academy and enter code: 319338

Along with sleep, other aspects of physical health are important in preparing for a test. Good nutrition is vital for good brain function. Sugary foods and drinks may give a burst of energy but this burst is followed by a crash, both physically and emotionally. Instead, fuel your body with protein and vitamin-rich foods.

Also, drink plenty of water. Dehydration can lead to headaches and exhaustion, especially if your brain is already under stress from the rigors of the test. Particularly if your test is a long one, drink water during the breaks. And if possible, take an energy-boosting snack to eat between sections.

> **Review Video: How Diet Can Affect your Mood**
> Visit mometrix.com/academy and enter code: 624317

Along with sleep and diet, a third important part of physical health is exercise. Maintaining a steady workout schedule is helpful, but even taking 5-minute study breaks to walk can help get your blood pumping faster and clear your head. Exercise also releases endorphins, which contribute to a positive feeling and can help combat test anxiety.

When you nurture your physical health, you are also contributing to your mental health. If your body is healthy, your mind is much more likely to be healthy as well. So take time to rest, nourish your body with healthy food and water, and get moving as much as possible. Taking these physical steps will make you stronger and more able to take the mental steps necessary to overcome test anxiety.

Mental Steps for Beating Test Anxiety

Working on the mental side of test anxiety can be more challenging, but as with the physical side, there are clear steps you can take to overcome it. As mentioned earlier, test anxiety often stems from lack of preparation, so the obvious solution is to prepare for the test. Effective studying may be the most important weapon you have for beating test anxiety, but you can and should employ several other mental tools to combat fear.

First, boost your confidence by reminding yourself of past success—tests or projects that you aced. If you're putting as much effort into preparing for this test as you did for those, there's no reason you should expect to fail here. Work hard to prepare; then trust your preparation.

Second, surround yourself with encouraging people. It can be helpful to find a study group, but be sure that the people you're around will encourage a positive attitude. If you spend time with others who are anxious or cynical, this will only contribute to your own anxiety. Look for others who are motivated to study hard from a desire to succeed, not from a fear of failure.

Third, reward yourself. A test is physically and mentally tiring, even without anxiety, and it can be helpful to have something to look forward to. Plan an activity following the test, regardless of the outcome, such as going to a movie or getting ice cream.

When you are taking the test, if you find yourself beginning to feel anxious, remind yourself that you know the material. Visualize successfully completing the test. Then take a few deep, relaxing breaths and return to it. Work through the questions carefully but with confidence, knowing that you are capable of succeeding.

Developing a healthy mental approach to test taking will also aid in other areas of life. Test anxiety affects more than just the actual test—it can be damaging to your mental health and even contribute to depression. It's important to beat test anxiety before it becomes a problem for more than testing.

Review Video: Test Anxiety and Depression
Visit mometrix.com/academy and enter code: 904704

Study Strategy

Being prepared for the test is necessary to combat anxiety, but what does being prepared look like? You may study for hours on end and still not feel prepared. What you need is a strategy for test prep. The next few pages outline our recommended steps to help you plan out and conquer the challenge of preparation.

STEP 1: SCOPE OUT THE TEST

Learn everything you can about the format (multiple choice, essay, etc.) and what will be on the test. Gather any study materials, course outlines, or sample exams that may be available. Not only will this help you to prepare, but knowing what to expect can help to alleviate test anxiety.

STEP 2: MAP OUT THE MATERIAL

Look through the textbook or study guide and make note of how many chapters or sections it has. Then divide these over the time you have. For example, if a book has 15 chapters and you have five days to study, you need to cover three chapters each day. Even better, if you have the time, leave an extra day at the end for overall review after you have gone through the material in depth.

If time is limited, you may need to prioritize the material. Look through it and make note of which sections you think you already have a good grasp on, and which need review. While you are studying, skim quickly through the familiar sections and take more time on the challenging parts. Write out your plan so you don't get lost as you go. Having a written plan also helps you feel more in control of the study, so anxiety is less likely to arise from feeling overwhelmed at the amount to cover.

STEP 3: GATHER YOUR TOOLS

Decide what study method works best for you. Do you prefer to highlight in the book as you study and then go back over the highlighted portions? Or do you type out notes of the important information? Or is it helpful to make flashcards that you can carry with you? Assemble the pens, index cards, highlighters, post-it notes, and any other materials you may need so you won't be distracted by getting up to find things while you study.

If you're having a hard time retaining the information or organizing your notes, experiment with different methods. For example, try color-coding by subject with colored pens, highlighters, or post-it notes. If you learn better by hearing, try recording yourself reading your notes so you can listen while in the car, working out, or simply sitting at your desk. Ask a friend to quiz you from your flashcards, or try teaching someone the material to solidify it in your mind.

STEP 4: CREATE YOUR ENVIRONMENT

It's important to avoid distractions while you study. This includes both the obvious distractions like visitors and the subtle distractions like an uncomfortable chair (or a too-comfortable couch that makes you want to fall asleep). Set up the best study environment possible: good lighting and a comfortable work area. If background music helps you focus, you may want to turn it on, but otherwise keep the room quiet. If you are using a computer to take notes, be sure you don't have any other windows open, especially applications like social media, games, or anything else that could distract you. Silence your phone and turn off notifications. Be sure to keep water close by so you stay hydrated while you study (but avoid unhealthy drinks and snacks).

Also, take into account the best time of day to study. Are you freshest first thing in the morning? Try to set aside some time then to work through the material. Is your mind clearer in the afternoon or evening? Schedule your study session then. Another method is to study at the same time of day that

163

you will take the test, so that your brain gets used to working on the material at that time and will be ready to focus at test time.

STEP 5: STUDY!

Once you have done all the study preparation, it's time to settle into the actual studying. Sit down, take a few moments to settle your mind so you can focus, and begin to follow your study plan. Don't give in to distractions or let yourself procrastinate. This is your time to prepare so you'll be ready to fearlessly approach the test. Make the most of the time and stay focused.

Of course, you don't want to burn out. If you study too long you may find that you're not retaining the information very well. Take regular study breaks. For example, taking five minutes out of every hour to walk briskly, breathing deeply and swinging your arms, can help your mind stay fresh.

As you get to the end of each chapter or section, it's a good idea to do a quick review. Remind yourself of what you learned and work on any difficult parts. When you feel that you've mastered the material, move on to the next part. At the end of your study session, briefly skim through your notes again.

But while review is helpful, cramming last minute is NOT. If at all possible, work ahead so that you won't need to fit all your study into the last day. Cramming overloads your brain with more information than it can process and retain, and your tired mind may struggle to recall even previously learned information when it is overwhelmed with last-minute study. Also, the urgent nature of cramming and the stress placed on your brain contribute to anxiety. You'll be more likely to go to the test feeling unprepared and having trouble thinking clearly.

So don't cram, and don't stay up late before the test, even just to review your notes at a leisurely pace. Your brain needs rest more than it needs to go over the information again. In fact, plan to finish your studies by noon or early afternoon the day before the test. Give your brain the rest of the day to relax or focus on other things, and get a good night's sleep. Then you will be fresh for the test and better able to recall what you've studied.

STEP 6: TAKE A PRACTICE TEST

Many courses offer sample tests, either online or in the study materials. This is an excellent resource to check whether you have mastered the material, as well as to prepare for the test format and environment.

Check the test format ahead of time: the number of questions, the type (multiple choice, free response, etc.), and the time limit. Then create a plan for working through them. For example, if you have 30 minutes to take a 60-question test, your limit is 30 seconds per question. Spend less time on the questions you know well so that you can take more time on the difficult ones.

If you have time to take several practice tests, take the first one open book, with no time limit. Work through the questions at your own pace and make sure you fully understand them. Gradually work up to taking a test under test conditions: sit at a desk with all study materials put away and set a timer. Pace yourself to make sure you finish the test with time to spare and go back to check your answers if you have time.

After each test, check your answers. On the questions you missed, be sure you understand why you missed them. Did you misread the question (tests can use tricky wording)? Did you forget the information? Or was it something you hadn't learned? Go back and study any shaky areas that the practice tests reveal.

164

Taking these tests not only helps with your grade, but also aids in combating test anxiety. If you're already used to the test conditions, you're less likely to worry about it, and working through tests until you're scoring well gives you a confidence boost. Go through the practice tests until you feel comfortable, and then you can go into the test knowing that you're ready for it.

Test Tips

On test day, you should be confident, knowing that you've prepared well and are ready to answer the questions. But aside from preparation, there are several test day strategies you can employ to maximize your performance.

First, as stated before, get a good night's sleep the night before the test (and for several nights before that, if possible). Go into the test with a fresh, alert mind rather than staying up late to study.

Try not to change too much about your normal routine on the day of the test. It's important to eat a nutritious breakfast, but if you normally don't eat breakfast at all, consider eating just a protein bar. If you're a coffee drinker, go ahead and have your normal coffee. Just make sure you time it so that the caffeine doesn't wear off right in the middle of your test. Avoid sugary beverages, and drink enough water to stay hydrated but not so much that you need a restroom break 10 minutes into the test. If your test isn't first thing in the morning, consider going for a walk or doing a light workout before the test to get your blood flowing.

Allow yourself enough time to get ready, and leave for the test with plenty of time to spare so you won't have the anxiety of scrambling to arrive in time. Another reason to be early is to select a good seat. It's helpful to sit away from doors and windows, which can be distracting. Find a good seat, get out your supplies, and settle your mind before the test begins.

When the test begins, start by going over the instructions carefully, even if you already know what to expect. Make sure you avoid any careless mistakes by following the directions.

Then begin working through the questions, pacing yourself as you've practiced. If you're not sure on an answer, don't spend too much time on it, and don't let it shake your confidence. Either skip it and come back later, or eliminate as many wrong answers as possible and guess among the remaining ones. Don't dwell on these questions as you continue—put them out of your mind and focus on what lies ahead.

Be sure to read all of the answer choices, even if you're sure the first one is the right answer. Sometimes you'll find a better one if you keep reading. But don't second-guess yourself if you do immediately know the answer. Your gut instinct is usually right. Don't let test anxiety rob you of the information you know.

If you have time at the end of the test (and if the test format allows), go back and review your answers. Be cautious about changing any, since your first instinct tends to be correct, but make sure you didn't misread any of the questions or accidentally mark the wrong answer choice. Look over any you skipped and make an educated guess.

At the end, leave the test feeling confident. You've done your best, so don't waste time worrying about your performance or wishing you could change anything. Instead, celebrate the successful completion of this test. And finally, use this test to learn how to deal with anxiety even better next time.

Review Video: 5 Tips to Beat Test Anxiety
Visit mometrix.com/academy and enter code: 570656

Important Qualification

Not all anxiety is created equal. If your test anxiety is causing major issues in your life beyond the classroom or testing center, or if you are experiencing troubling physical symptoms related to your anxiety, it may be a sign of a serious physiological or psychological condition. If this sounds like your situation, we strongly encourage you to seek professional help.

Thank You

We at Mometrix would like to extend our heartfelt thanks to you, our friend and patron, for allowing us to play a part in your journey. It is a privilege to serve people from all walks of life who are unified in their commitment to building the best future they can for themselves.

The preparation you devote to these important testing milestones may be the most valuable educational opportunity you have for making a real difference in your life. We encourage you to put your heart into it—that feeling of succeeding, overcoming, and yes, conquering will be well worth the hours you've invested.

We want to hear your story, your struggles and your successes, and if you see any opportunities for us to improve our materials so we can help others even more effectively in the future, please share that with us as well. **The team at Mometrix would be absolutely thrilled to hear from you!** So please, send us an email (support@mometrix.com) and let's stay in touch.

> **If you'd like some additional help, check out these other resources we offer for your exam:**
> **http://mometrixflashcards.com/CMC**

Additional Bonus Material

Due to our efforts to try to keep this book to a manageable length, we've created a link that will give you access to all of your additional bonus material.

Please visit **https://www.mometrix.com/bonus948/cmc** to access the information.